the
tortoise
effect

making progress in spite of pain

JUANITA M. CLENDANIEL

ISBN 978-1-7355883-2-2 (Softcover Book)
ISBN 978-1-7355883-3-9 (eBook)

Printed in the United States of America

Pubished by Publish & GO Press—Houston, Texas
www.publishandgo.com

PUBLISH & GO PRESS
HOUSTON

Contents

Dedication

I would like to dedicate this book first, to my family for their unconditional love, and to all of my doctors for sharing their expertise with me to help me put the pieces of the puzzle together in my life so I could keep moving forward.

Acknowledgements

_____

Thank you to Father God for His continued faithfulness in my life throughout this journey.

My mother, Myrtle Clendaniel, for wanting the best for me and taking me to my many doctor's appointments through the years. To my brother, Herbie Clendaniel, for letting me recoup at his house more than once as well as keeping me company and making me laugh. Joanna Hunt for your amazing coaching skills, patience and encouragement for me to get it down and "write, write, write." Dr. Naim and Dr. Hakeem Collins for encouraging me to write and telling me that my audience will come. To all those who assisted me in any way through prayer and encouragement every step of the way. I have the best family and friends that anyone could ask for. To my worship family at Destiny Christian Church thank you for your love and understanding.

Cover design and layout: Chris Boyer

Author photo: Laura Navarre

CHAPTER ONE

Journey With Pain

"No temptation has overtaken you except what is common to mankind. And God is faithful; he will not let you be tempted beyond what you can bear. But when you are tempted, he will also provide a way out so that you can endure it."

1 CORINTHIANS 10:13

No one asks for a life of pain. Yet, my journey with pain began almost from the beginning. Yes, as a baby. I blocked a lot of it out but when I was 42 years old, I learned something shocking from my doctor—not about my present health condition, but about my childhood.

That particular summer, I was in a week long dance intensive which lasted about two hours every day. Usually a dance class lasts 45 minutes to an hour. A dance intensive means that it lasts longer. Summer intensives are usually all day. I go to the ballet class only. You see, my whole life, I've loved dance and as an adult, I became a teacher part time teaching music theater to the dancers, voice/piano lessons and substituting when needed. Because I had been dancing for so many years, I didn't feel the need to stretch before the sessions (who does). I had a great summer dance intensive that year. I felt really strong and flexible. The dancers have about a three-week break from dance classes in August. After two weeks I thought I had better start stretching. When I got home one afternoon after a particularly challenging day, I was pretty sore and stiff. I have a ballet barre (portable handrail that you use for support while working on flexibility and balance) in my home and decided to do some stretching to help relax my body. I walked over to the barre as I had done a thousand times before. However, the moment I lifted my leg up to place my foot on the barre, I heard a loud pop in my knee and felt the most excruciating pain. I immediately called a friend who recommended that I go see an orthopedist, Dr. Reisman. I was able to get an appointment right away and during the evaluation, Dr. Reisman studied the way I moved with great curiosity. He asked me all about my health history which is quite extensive. For some reason, I always seem to have issues on the right side of my body, even though my injury this time was on my left leg. For example, I had eye surgery to shorten the opening of my right eyelid, my right hip is tilted inward, my right leg is hyper extended which has caused balance issues my whole life. Even my right ovary is abnormal. I had an ultrasound one time and the technician said to me, "I can't find your right ovary, it's bent out of place."

I told all of this to the doctor and he asked me, "Do you know what happened while you were being born?"

I thought, what kind of question is that?

"No, I actually don't remember my birth. I can probably guess that the doctor held me up and slapped me on my butt. At least that's what always happens in the movies." I replied slightly sarcastically.

He didn't flinch, chuckle, or even crack a smile. Then he said something to me that I will never forget. "Something happened to you when you were born and you are dealing with it now as an adult. It's like you have a slight case of cerebral palsy."

Cerebral palsy??!! What?

His hypothesis about my birth was troubling to say the least. How could I not know something like that? As he continued to talk, I couldn't focus on any of his words. He said my injury was likely related to a weakness in my right side and I was overcompensating and stressing the left side to the point of tearing my hamstring. He gave me some pain killers and sent me on my way.

I immediately went home to talk with my mother who was staying with me during this time. I told her what the doctor said. She just looked at me somberly.

"Yes, that's what they told me when you were born. They thought it was cerebral palsy." What? I was completely stunned. How could she know this and not tell me after all these years? She went on to explain that something happened during my birth as I was passing through the birth canal. I could hardly hear her words. It all seemed so surreal. I was too overwhelmed to even ask her why she never told me until that point.

Later on, when we were able to talk more about it, she told me that she and my father didn't want me to be defined or limited by a diagnosis, and I never was.

What I thought I knew about my childhood, begins when I was learning to walk. Around thirteen months old, my mother saw that I kept trying to walk but would constantly fall down, way more than other babies at that age. She watched me carefully and saw that it was because my right foot was not flat on the floor, something she never noticed until I tried to walk. Because my foot was naturally tilted out, I was having balance issues. Walking was a huge challenge.

My mom took me to my first podiatrist visit in Wilmington, Delaware. It was the first of many appointments throughout my childhood as my mom tried to find any answers so she could help me. Back in the early 60s, there weren't many specialists in Dover, Delaware, where we lived. We had to drive almost an hour from our home to the podiatrist's office. My earliest memories of traveling to the doctor always include images of those dreadful bridges we'd have to cross over, the St. George Bridge and the North Market Street Bridge. They were massive bridges with tall steel scaffolding and they frightened me as a young girl. Looking out the car window as we drove, seeing those bridges in the distance would give me an immediate pit in my stomach every time. Looking back, it's hard to say if the dread I felt was because of the bridges themselves, or because they signaled that we were getting close to another miserable doctor's appointment.

I blocked out those bridges and every memory of every doctor's appointment for many years. It wasn't until a strange phenomenon as an adult that the memories came back.

Once we got over the bridges, we were in the big city, or at least it seemed big compared to the one light town we lived in. Each visit, the doctor would check me over and tell me to walk up and down the hallway. I had to walk slowly down and back, and then on my toes down and back. He studied my movement carefully and checked my knee reflexes with a small rubber mallet. There were no x-ray machines at that time so the only way the doctor could determine what was wrong with my foot was by external observation. My mom asked if there were any exercises that she could do with me to help improve the condition of my foot. He told her no. Sadly, back in the early 60s, we did not have physical therapy or sports medicine like we do today.

Eventually, the fateful day came when the doctor prescribed a brace for me to wear every night and special laced shoes during the day. The goal of using a brace was to try to force my foot to straighten out so that it would be flat on the ground when I walked. In order to fulfill the doctor's recommendation, my mom had to go to a special shoe store and buy two pairs of high-top shoes to work with the brace. She then took them to a shoe repair shop where the cobbler put an insert on the side and inside of my shoe so that my foot would lay flat. These shoes were to be worn during the day. The second pair of shoes were bought for my right brace. Only one shoe was used. The cobbler attached the braces, one on each side of the heel of the shoe.

Wearing that brace was extremely painful and I had to wear it until I was 14 years old.

Yes, 14 years of my life, that brace taunted me and I hated it. I didn't want to wear it, but mom made sure that I did. When I would go to bed at night, she would holler to me in my room, "Juanita! Do you have your brace on?"

"Yes, mom!"

I hated that stupid brace and sometimes I would lie about wearing it. Somehow, she always knew. She would come in and check to make sure.

Through the night, while trying to sleep, my foot would just throb in pain, and then I would have to deal with the weight of that heavy brace hitting my other leg as I tossed and turned in my sleep. The struggle was real. I would constantly wake up in the night and I was always covered in bruises because of it.

The shoes that I wore during the day had to be laced high tops to support my ankles with arch supports inside my shoes. I hated wearing high-top shoes as a kid. None of the other kids were wearing them at the time, but now as an adult...ironically, I love them! One particular summer a couple of months after one of my surgeries, I wore high tops because my foot felt less pain than when I wore regular shoes. When I went to the podiatrist to have this checked, the high tops were supporting my foot by holding the bones together.

One day, my podiatrist finally opened an office in Dover, only 20 minutes from home. Less travel made everything easier. By this time, I had to go see him every six months. This new office was housed in the Armory, which was around The Green, a historical site where the troops in the 1700s would gather for battle. All the buildings in that area are red brick with marble steps that lead to a big heavy door. The musty smell of the building is still vivid in my mind to this day. The office was located down a staircase in the basement. Again, trips to the doctor were filled with emotion but yet, going to a place where troops gathered for battle was a constant reminder that I was in a battle against pain and dysfunction in my body. But like those soldiers, I put on a brave face and never allowed this challenge to hold me back.

I remember the last day we went to see the doctor. I didn't know it was the last visit at the time. But on that particular day, the doctor looked at my progress and wrote something down on his clipboard. Then he said to us, "Well, I've done all I can do. You don't really need to come visit me anymore." I was very confused and thought, "He's got to be kidding. But...I still limp...how can this be it?" I was so shocked and had a wave of emotion inside that felt like it was going to explode. We aren't done yet! Is there no cure for this? Isn't there some way to fix it? The words rolled around in my head but I couldn't get them out of my mouth before my mother quietly said, "Thank you." And that was it. We went home.

We never talked anymore about going to the doctors and I just remained incredibly self-conscious about walking. People would notice me limping and some would even ask me, "What happened?" "Nothing." I would say. I didn't want to talk about it. I just wanted to be normal.

JOURNEY WITH PAIN

CHAPTER TWO

Wanting Normal

"Trust in the Lord with all your heart and lean not on your own understanding; in all your ways submit to him, and he will make your paths straight."

PROVERBS 3:5-6

When I was young, I would always try to do things that I saw other young kids doing. I tried to ride a bike, but I just couldn't get the hang of it. My dad tried his best to teach me, but I was always the kid riding the tricycle. I just couldn't get my balance. In fact, I didn't learn to ride a bicycle until I was 13 years old. But, I finally did it! I always wanted to ice skate, but that too seemed impossible. We had a big pond in the back of our house and in the cold winters of Delaware, the pond would freeze over. One year, dad bought all of my siblings and I ice skates. My sisters and I were so excited to go out and ice skate. Of course, I tried so hard to skate, but I would always wobble and fall all over the place. No balance whatsoever. As much as I wanted to, I just couldn't do it. So instead, I would sit out on the side of the pond in a little red chair known as "the hospital." If anyone would fall, they would yell, "Hospital! Hospital!" and I was very faithful to come over and rescue them. The hospital was a very important job during skating season, so I was content to be the hospital, even if I never got to skate.

Right along those lines, another pastime of the Clendaniel sisters, was roller skating. We loved roll- er-skating and we were at the roller rink at least 5 times a week. This was a little better for me since roller skates are far more stable than ice skates. I was slow at first, but at least I could do it. I could never seem to figure out how to do a turn no matter how hard I tried. I worked really hard to finally be able to go backwards. I even took lessons, but balance was still an issue and seemed to be my weakness for every activity.

My favorite activity of all was dancing. Our family would all get together on Saturday nights and watch The Lawrence Welk Show on TV. We loved Bobby and Cissy! They made dancing look so easy and graceful and I wanted so badly to be able to dance like that. I would sit mesmerized watch- ing them and when I wasn't watching them, I was dream- ing about dancing. Every time I would think of that show, I would just start dancing, no matter where I was. I would be playing outside and then just start dancing around as if I were a pro and the cameras were all on me. But then I would quickly snap back to reality anytime a car would pass by. I was always so embarrassed and self-conscience. My whole life, my movements had been analyzed by doctors. I knew at a young age that I had a "unique" walk and I just didn't want to be watched anymore.

As a teenager, I learned some different types of dancing that had less footwork and more hip work, which my mother really hated. My sisters and I would watch American Bandstand and The Steel Pier Show. We loved the music and jumping around and having fun shaking our bodies to the beat. Mom would hear us giggling and making a commotion in the living room and she would holler from the kitchen, "Are you girls dancing in there?"

"No, mom!"

"Then why are you all out of breath?" mom asked.

Busted!

In spite of the limitations I had in my body, my spirit never felt limited. However, there was a constant struggle between who I wanted to be and what was possible because of my physical dysfunction.

All throughout my childhood, I had this recurring dream about a huge ship. It had thick black ropes and tall sails. It reminded me of one of Christopher Columbus' ships. For some reason, the ship always gave me a bad feeling. It was enormous and daunting, towering over me. I would often wake up from this dream startled and scared. I couldn't understand why I was dreaming about this ship. I had never been on a boat or ship before. Was the dream trying to tell me something? I never told my mom or anybody about this, but I would dream it several times a month for many years, until I was almost 20 years old.

In my 20s, I attended college with a double major in business administration and music education. Because of my foot and balance issue, I had a lot of sprained ankles which meant being on crutches a lot. On my good days without crutches, I was still limping which gave me extremely tight hip flexors and caused a cycle of pain and stiffness. I was, however, faithful to stretch every day and did aerobics with my sisters which helped a lot. My sisters and I were always silly when we would get together and we would laugh at ourselves and have a good workout!

In college, I was involved in band and choir ensembles. I love to sing and play the piano. This commitment required traveling by bus to regional concerts from time to time. One time, we had a concert scheduled in a hotel in the city of Wilmington, Delaware—which I had no recollection of ever being there at this point. On the day of the event, everyone was on the bus having a great time talking, sharing, and anticipating the concert. I was laughing and looking out the window when the bus took a turn and I couldn't believe what I saw. Right there before my eyes was the very picture I had seen in my dream over and over again for almost 20 years. I saw the cables and what looked to be a massive ship, exactly like the one in my dreams. Except, it wasn't a ship, it was a bridge...over...water. What is this? I was thinking. I've never been here before. Why am I seeing this? Why have I been dreaming this for years? My friend, who was sitting next to me kept asking, "Juanita, are you OK? What's wrong?" I was just sitting there in shock and disbelief. I kept saying, "Oh my God. Oh My God. What

I'm looking at is what I've been dreaming about all these years."

The band played at the hotel and returned to the college campus in Dover, Delaware. When I arrived home, it was very late and no one at my house was awake, so I had some time alone with my thoughts. The next morning when I woke up, I walked out of my room and straight to find my mother.

"Mom, have I ever been over the North Market Street Bridge in Wilmington?"

"Yes. Yes, you have." She replied.

"I have? When?"

My mother told me about going to the podiatrist's office off the North Street Market Bridge when I was little. Then I told her about my reoccurring dream. In that moment, it was like there was a puzzle in my brain and the pieces started coming together. The imprint of the bridges and the fear that I experienced was so real and it wouldn't be resolved until many years later after receiving counseling. But it's almost like something inside me was saying, "It's time to sail away from those memories, the pain, the difficulty, and the fear. It's time to sail into the future."

I must admit, there is still a slight hesitation when going over bridges but not as severe once I understood that I had associated pain with bridges. I always ask anyone in the car with me to keep talking to me while driving over a bridge!

In 1995, I moved to Felton, Delaware. Before that, I spent a couple of years in Tulsa learning the music business and then moved back to be closer to family again. I began playing the piano in college and hoped to play at my church when I moved back home, but they already had a pianist. I believe strongly in serving in the church, I just didn't know what my involvement would be. I thought, "They dance." This small voice answered, "You used to when you were younger." I had forgotten all about me dancing outside when I was a little girl.

My sister attended the same church and was part of the dance team that would join the worship services. Being on the dance team looked fun. I always loved dancing but I was so self-conscious still. One Sunday in the middle of the worship service, my sister leaned over to me and whispered, "Follow me!" Without hesitation, I fell into formation with the other dancers and followed the leader right up to the platform at the front of the church. I was having so much fun copying every move until the leader went down on one knee. "Ugh! I can't go down on one knee," I thought, "I'll never be able to get up!" I danced over to the side and hoped no one would see me. I wondered if anyone saw that I didn't go down on one knee.

I officially joined the dance team and learned to dance with streamers, flags, double flags and tambourines. Each Sunday, there was a different lead dancer assigned. If anyone on the dance team wanted to go on to the platform and dance, they were to make a signal to the leader who would let you know when you could go up. One Sunday, the dance leader pointed to me to go up on to the platform. I hadn't asked, she just picked me and I was so excited! I headed to the platform steps and started to jump up the steps, only to miss one and I tripped and fell on the steps. My left knee hit the edge of the step and hurt like crazy. But my pride hurt even worse. I was beyond embarrassed and just froze right there for a second. Thankfully the stairs were off to the side and people were standing and engaged in worship. But I was in so much pain. I thought to myself, "Boy, this stinks." I quickly mustered up the courage to hobble up on to the platform and still performed something with my streamer even though it was totally tangled up when I first got up there. Fortunately, no one knew that I had fallen but people were asking me later about why my flag was tangled up.

Dancing

As I was turning 39 in the summer of 1999, I decided that it was time to take some formal dance lessons. I asked some of my friends if they wanted to take dance classes with me. It shouldn't be too hard, right? We could have fun together while learning like we do in the dance groups at church. Besides, we will have more knowledge and better skills to help us with dance specials.

The only issue was that the local dance studio only had one beginning level class which was for all ages. So, we would be starting at the beginning with the little kids, ages 5-6 years old, but we would work up in the levels. My friends all said to me, "Are you crazy? I am not taking dance classes with little kids." Oh boy! I couldn't get any-one to take dance classes with me. I didn't let this become a bummer. I would take dance classes by myself. So that's what I did.

The day of the first class, I was excited and nervous. I arrived and saw all the young girls in their pink leotards and ballet slippers. I thought to myself, "What are you do-ing? An adult taking classes with young kids." But I loved to dance so much that within a few minutes, I was lost in learning the movements. After the first class, I began learning the terminology and techniques.

I enjoyed learning ballet, social dance, tap/jazz, and jazz. I was thrilled to be doing something that I always want-ed to do. I worked hard and a lot of times I would wake in the morning and my body would feel so stiff. Over time, I learned how to keep going while experiencing foot spasms and a tight back. Ballet was very good for my body but it took about six months before I could dance without pain in my back.

Walking out of the studio was better than walking in. This was a good thing. I remember buying and reading a ballet book entitled, "The Joffrey Ballet School's Ballet-Fit" by Dena Simone Moss and Allison Kyle Leopold. This helped me as an adult ballet dancer. The book stated, "As long as you continue to take class regularly, you cannot not im-prove. Just keep in mind that in ballet, progress is always gradual; it's the nature of the art." My thoughts held on to this statement and it fueled my determination.

After a year, I had the opportunity to go to a Christian dance summer intensive for a week. The dance classes were on hard floor surfaces and by the second day, I could feel pain in my foot. Yes, I had an injury. However, I kept dancing in spite of it for the rest of the week. It was wonderful and we were presented with a lot of awesome information. After the intensive, I went home and continued with my ballet classes. The pain in my foot became more severe. After one class, I approached the ballet teacher and she suggested that I go see a podiatrist. Reluctantly, I went and they told me I had a pinched nerve. Thank goodness they ruled out a stress fracture!

The rest of the summer was filled with doctor's visits and at-home therapy and stretches. Eventually, the doctor evaluated me and said that I would be fine. I was released from his care. However, my foot was still in pain. I had to go to another podiatrist. Off to Wilmington I would go. I found a podiatrist who specializes in sports medicine and dancer's feet. I was finally on the right track, at last. All of my podiatrists were wonderful up to this point and helped me find my way to health and I'm so grateful. But this doctor seemed to be more specialized in sports medicine which is what I needed. He helped me recover from the pinched nerve and back to ballet class I went!

There was always such a calmness that came over me while taking class. I loved the beautiful music. I stayed focus on my goals to find balance, lengthen my legs, and increase my range of motion. This was my form of exercise and I found it thoroughly enjoyable and relaxing. If you call stretching your body into pretzel forms relaxing. Some people don't. However, I do.

Move through late 2003, I found myself doing donkey kicks and spider walks in a jazz class only to have my big toe grind into the floor. This was done two minutes before class would be over. Bummer! However, that didn't stop me from going to my next class, which was a performance class. Actually, I didn't even think of not going to my next dance class. My foot was tingly and painful. Now I know something had happened to my foot. My podiatrist (yes, you guessed it, up in Wilmington) gave me a cortisone shot and scheduled my first bunionectomy for December, 2003.

The podiatrist told me not to dance on my foot for a week. I asked if I could dance in "The Nutcracker." He said, "Of course." I told him that "The Nutcracker" ballet auditions were Saturday, the next day. I will always remember him whipping around and saying, "and you will not be there." Oh boy. After the lecture and the trip back from Wilmington to Dover (an hour), I stopped in to the dance studio. I talked with the Artistic Director. She told me to come to auditions but sit on the sidelines. There would be no dancing for me that day. She told me to come back the following week and dance with the callbacks. I was very excited to not have missed out on the opportunity to play "A rat." The dancers were telling me that the auditions for the Rats were called. I told them that I couldn't audition today but will be with callbacks the next week. The dancers knew that I wanted to be "A Rat" really bad that year. I had been an adult Party Person for two years and Mrs. Stahlbaum for two years. So, I really wanted to be a Rat. The Rat had a lot of fun on stage. Yes, the part was mine! Yes, I had a lot of fun! What a great experience.

Monday, the next day after The Nutcracker, I drove with my mom to Wilmington for the surgery. This would be the day after the five performances of "The Nutcracker." The surgery went well. There were no problems nor complications. I felt great. Mom and I went out to eat at a restaurant before going home. The medication was kicking in. Why not eat? There would be a week off from work to heal. After that time back to work with my mom being my chauffeur driving back and forth to work.

The first day back to work was when there was a co-worker stating that she hoped that I didn't expect her to get things for me. OK! Welcome back to work! That afternoon, there was a fire drill at the company. Crutches here we go! When I tried to get out of the building, people were not even holding the door for me. No one seemed to see that I was hobbling while using crutches. OK! Hello self...welcome back to the real world.

I had been dealing with plantar fasciitis on my right foot. I felt the fibers ripping from the bottom of my foot when I was at a rehearsal with the African Dancing and Drumming Group, Sankofa. I was glad that I finished the dance and then went to the sidelines. Back to the podiatrists I went. There would be cortisone treatments, physical therapy for stretching and help. The treatments were helping my right foot. Then got plantar fasciitis on the left foot. Getting cortisone treatments then physical therapy for stretching and help. Do you see a pattern here? As time went by, there would be several Excellence Shock Wave Therapy treatments done to the right foot. These treatments had some relief for a while and then something else always seemed to pop up. Lord help me! Why was I always getting injured with my feet?

During one of those injuries I was a dancer with an African Dancing and Drumming group, Sankofa. I was the one warming up the dancers. I would also go to the performances and make sure everyone had their costumes and was ready to go. It was 2 days a week with 3 hours for each session. This form of dance was very freeing. Definitely the opposite of the strict dance form of ballet. I went to a performance with a group of dancers and drummers at Swarthmore College in Pennsylvania. It was a great performance. At the end, the performing dancers went through the audience and picked people to come and dance on the stage. Of course, I was picked. I seem to never be able to hide in the crowd. I told them that I was injured. They said that would be no problem. They told me to go up on stage anyway. OK. So, I did. My foot got warmed up and I was enjoying myself. Was my foot in pain. Yep. After I got home, I iced it and it was good to go.

The second bunionectomy was done June 2012. There was a rod, and screws put in my foot to hold my bones in place. This would be a couple of months non-weight bearing. I stayed at my brother's house until I felt comfortable to be on my own. The doctor prescribed Percocet. Normally this would put people to sleep. Ha! Not me. I would be out for an hour and then wide awake for the whole night. I was at my brother's house for a few weeks until I felt that I could go home to my house.

While transitioning from boot to sneakers, there was a feeling of getting stronger and walking better. My doctor told me to keep working my foot and start jumping little by little. "Your foot will be fine as long as the bones fused together," my doctor said in passing. So that's what I did. I started walking on my foot longer and jumping a little. After about a month or so I felt more pain in my foot. Something wasn't right. I was thinking this pain would work itself out. As a dancer, you work through the pain. That's what I did. However, a person at church came to me and asked what has happened to my foot. They stated that I had been walking better a few weeks earlier. I realized that I had to go back to the podiatrist.

The podiatrist had already scheduled a surgery for me in January 14, 2013; however, when we met in December, the procedures to be performed at the surgery was changed. I would have the screws taken out and put back in, with a plate, and a bone graft to glue my bones back together. My doctor was also putting a bone stimulator in my foot to help the bones heal. I told him that if he needed to scrap bone from a cadaver to make sure they were an active, Zumba, ballet-kind of person. He laughed at that statement. I personally didn't want to use bone coming from a couch potato. The wire that was attached to the bone stimulator was right above a nerve on the top of my foot. I had to learn how to tie my shoes in a different way than normal.

The next surgery would be the following year, July 7, 2014, in which my podiatrist would be taking the bone stimulator out of my foot. After the surgery, he stated that the wire from the bone stimulator just came out with a little pull. He also stated that this does not happen. I explained that I was having the Graston technique done by my chiropractor. This would be why the wire from the bone stimulator was not attached to my ligaments. Graston is when tools are used to scrape across ligaments to release adhesions and to help increase blood flow and restore movement and flexibility. Because of this procedure, the wire was easily pulled out. However, while Graston is being done it is painful. I remember singing Italian Arias to my doctor!

WANTING NORMAL

CHAPTER THREE

Learning to Live Life to the Fullest

*"Have mercy upon me, O LORD; for I am weak: O LORD,
heal me; for my bones are troubled."*

PSALM 6:2 – KJB

As you can see, I am an expert on pain. This was not one of my goals in life; however, it has become my experience. Even as I write, there are still more instances coming to mind that I had forgotten. Like when I sprained both of my ankles during roller skating lessons. When I started taking lessons, the instructor told me that I had the perfect back for roller skating. Who knew? She said, "Don't let anyone talk you out of roller skating." I might have the perfect back; however, it takes more than just your back to land jumps. And I certainly couldn't master four-point turns. The fact that I didn't have the perfect feet for roller skating was not really a surprise for me. I had two left feet. The last straw was when I was skating at the roller rink and everyone was to go under the limbo stick. I did go under the limbo stick while my body went one way and my feet went the opposite. Ouch! I heard pops and had to be helped off the floor. Great, two sprained ankles! Needless to say, I gave up roller skating.

Have you ever seen the episode of The Office entitled, "The Injury" where Michael burned his foot on the grill and had to use crutches? Bless his heart. He always seemed to be in the way of everybody around him. He was trying to help and felt so unappreciated. I first saw this episode when I was four months non-weight bearing, meaning I myself was on crutches. I laughed until I cried. During this time, I was off work and bored. So, I don't know if the show was really that funny or if I was laughing because I could relate to what he was going through. He thought he was disabled. It was the funniest thing I had ever seen. He was so awkward on the crutches. He could barely get in and out of the car and was struggling the entire show. He just wanted to do the things he normally would do; however, he was injured. The reality is that when you are injured, you simply can't do what you normally do with the same speed as when you are not injured. Injuries make you slow down!

A torn hamstring is another obstacle that I had to deal with. One time, I was stretching in a hot studio which would normally be great because dancers become more flexible when stretching in heat; however, I overstretched and felt a pop! Moments before the pop, I was talking with my best friend, who is also a dancer, showing her how close my split-straddle-split was to the floor. I was very excited to see that I only needed about one more inch for my legs to be parallel to the floor. "Watch this," I said to my friend. I went into my right split followed by my straddle followed by...pop! A jolt went through my leg. I was in such pain asking my friend to help me. She thought I was imitating someone at the studio. "I've never seen any dancer do that. Who are you imitating?" I kept saying, "Help me! Help me!" as I held my leg in excruciating pain. My friend was saying, "No one at the studio acts like that." I said, "I know. I need help." She then realized that I was injured and helped me up. "I need to get through this ballet class," I said to my friend. "Ballet class! You have a musical theater performance to get through after the ballet class. Even after this injury, which was a torn hamstring, I didn't miss my ballet class or the musical theater performance. Yes, I performed with the pain. Was it worth it? Yes, it was! Did I have to take pain medicine? Yes, I did. Did I look awkward? Maybe! I obviously was not 100% but did it! That's all that mattered to me.

Even though I've endured a lot of injuries through the years, I don't want anyone to feel sorry for me. These injuries have actually empowered me. Through these injuries I've learned that life will not pass me by. As long as I live, there will be a dream to fulfill. I'm never too old to try new things. Neither are you. Pain should not hold us down. There might be things needed for support, a brace, compression socks, knee brace, or the like but, there's always a way to have an active lifestyle.

It seemed the injuries were always coming one right after the other. Just when one thing was getting healed, it seemed that another injury was lurking around the corner. One time during a ballet summer intensive, I was very strong, went to class daily, stretched, and did what I had to do and had a very rewarding time in ballet class. My feet felt strong and that was a great feeling. I was also finding my balance, which is important in ballet class. Just afterward, around August, I wasn't doing any classes and it was time to rest my body with light stretching which is precisely when I popped my knee. I went to an orthopedist to explain what happened and it turned into a laughing spree. I told him that I was at the barre and my knee popped, when I was straightening my leg. He heard, "I was dancing on the bar and my knee popped." He wanted to know why I was on the bar—and if I was drinking. I expressed to him that I was not on the bar I was at the barre. "We are talking ballet here," but he had no clue. Needless to say, he was educated in ballet terminology that day.

With every injury I would ask God, "Why me? Why now? What did I do to have this pain come to my life?" I would always feel like it was a personal attack on me. Since I am a Christian, I can definitely say that it is a personal attack on me. Good vs. evil. Sometimes we have to look at the big picture instead of looking at the daily situations. "But God chose the foolish things of the world to shame the wise; God chose the weak things of the world to shame the strong (1 Corinthians 1:27, Bible Hub). Sometimes it's not about us in the physical world but in the spiritual world. "For we wrestle not against flesh and blood, but against principalities, against powers, against the rulers of the darkness of this world, against spiritual wickedness in high places"

(Ephesians 6:12, KJV).

When you are in constant pain it is very crippling. Your main goal is to get relief. You feel like crying out, "Can someone help me out here, please!" Have you ever felt this way? One particular time, when I was four months non-weight bearing (on crutches) my foot kept going into a spasm. I watched the clock to see how often this spasm happened. I remember clearly that I started observing the time starting at 10:30 p.m. I noticed that my foot spasm happened every minute and lasted for five seconds. Here it comes, 10:31. Here it comes, 10:32. I observed this until 4:30 a.m. Yep! Sure enough! Five seconds for every minute. Needless to say, sleep was not happening. When I called the doctor the next day, with this new medical data that was collected, he stated that he did not implant any timing device in me. He felt that since I was a music teacher, I was merely sensitive to the rhythm.

I also learned from one of my doctors, since my body did not have any distractions while trying to get some sleep, the pain was more severe. She stated that during the day, my body was focused on watching the television, talking to people on the telephone, thumbing through Facebook, listening to music, etc. When trying to sleep, there was nothing to distract my body from the pain. Therefore, my body was focused on one thing: Pain! Great! Me and pain all night long!

Pain is Personal

I've heard that this should not be taken personally; however, how can pain not be taken personally? Please don't ever tell someone that pain is only in their head. It's not, and it affects every part of your life. Yes, pain is very personal. When you are attacked with pain it will make you sit up and take notice. Pain tells you that something is wrong. Pain tells you that some area needs attention. Unless you deal with the pain, it will still linger on. For me, I had to take medication, which I hated. My body didn't react to medication the way it should. But, when my foot was throbbing, something had to give so I could get relief from the pain. Even though the side effect of prescription medication made me feel loopy. Anytime I felt down and out, or weak and overwhelmed, I had to remind myself that my strength comes from the Lord.

Gaining as much knowledge as I could about my situation also helped me with the healing process. I was able to understand how my whole being was affected by injuries. For example, I understand that when there is a problem with your feet, there will also be problems with your knees, hips, and back. Your feet are the foundation for your body. If your feet are out of alignment, your whole body will be out of alignment. Not only did I study how my body is affected physically, I studied the spiritual parallels too. I prayed and asked God, "God, what is going on with me spiritually?" As I was dealing with my physical foundation, I felt that God was dealing with my spiritual foundation and bringing my whole life into alignment. I realized that things that I thought were important at one time, are not really that important at all. I had to learn, and I'm still learning how to slow down and enjoy the moment. When you're injured, nothing happens very quickly, so I was sort of forced into learning how to stop and smell the roses, if you will.

The physical and mental limitations are also something that I had to take into account. I wouldn't be able to do the activities that I regularly did. Before the surgery, my activities included Zumba, weight lifting, elliptical machines, walking, Nike Challenges, Fitbit Challenges and dance classes. As you see, I had an active lifestyle! Without being active, I would be stuck at home by myself, gaining weight and dealing with high blood pressure. This was a very daunting feeling. I didn't like the feeling of being dependent on others as well.

When I was four months non-weight bearing all my independence was taken away. No driving because the surgeries were on my right foot. Thank goodness I had my mother to rely on to transport me to and from doctor's appointments, running errands, and church. My mom had six kids and was a stay at home mother. Before the surgery, I was traveling the roads to ballet classes, music seminars, concerts, meetings, etc. I knew where all the fast food stores were and what type of food they had and where I could find an ATM machine if I needed money. I would just go, go, go! After the surgery, when I was non-weight bearing, I had to rely on my mom for driving; she had no idea where my favorite food places were, didn't know what they had and had never used an ATM card. Frustration was quite the feeling when I knew where everything was; however, my mom had never been in these stores before. I wanted a chocolate chip cookie. My mom said, "Nita, there are no chocolate chip cookies." Oh boy! I climbed out of the car, took my crutches, hobbled over where they were and BAM! no chocolate chip cookies! I just wanted a chocolate chip cookie but had to settle for something else. Of course, my attitude wasn't the nicest either. Sorry, mom!

The thought of being immobile scared me and there was a huge learning curve with the crutches for sure. My hands would hurt all the time while using them even though my brother wrapped the handles with towels for cushions. Going down steps was easier than going up. I had to kneel and crawl while pulling myself up in order to go up the stairs. I didn't worry much about how silly I looked when I was just with my mom, however, climbing the stairs at the church platform to play the piano was a different scenario. I would put my crutches on the top steps, and crawl up, then I would pull myself up onto the piano stool. I could not push down the sustaining pedal with my right foot, so I had to twist my body so that my left foot could hold down the sustaining pedal. This was a very awkward position for me.

I would tell the worship team not to look over toward me while I was playing the piano. It was all such work for me, from getting onto the platform, then playing the piano, and trying to focus on the music—which was hopefully in the right order—and then I had to not focus on the pain in my throbbing foot. God bless the worship team who was so supportive through all of this. Very often I was frustrated about it all. It just didn't seem fair. I never complained to anyone; however, God and I would have long talks. How do you expect me to be up here and usher people into praise and worship when I really feel like crap? Why couldn't someone else be up here? Why did I have to deal with this pain in front of everybody?

When praise and worship were over, I would grab one crutch and give the other to a band member to hold for me so I could grab the banister with the other hand, go down the stairs and then get my other crutch at the bottom. I would hop back to the bathroom and then go back to my seat in the back of the church. I was always aware that people were staring during this whole display. What were people thinking about me? Maybe they were just glad that it wasn't them. I don't know. No one came to me to give their condolences for my present situation, which in hindsight was a good thing.

When God Spoke to Me

One day while talking with God, He said, "You know, it's not about you?"

I thought, "Well, you could have really fooled me, God. because I am the one injured here."

Then I turned to a scripture in the Bible, "And if the spirit of him who raised Jesus from the dead is living in you, he who raised Christ from the dead will also give life to your mortal bodies because of his Spirit who lives in you"

(Romans 8:11). There is definitely some raising up needed! Another passage in the Bible that really hit home, and proved God's point of view, "But we have this treasure in jars of clay to show that this all-surpassing power is from God and not from us. We are hard pressed on every side, but not crushed; perplexed, but not in despair, persecuted, but not abandoned; struck down, but not destroyed. We always carry around in our body the death of Jesus, so that the life of Jesus may also be revealed in our body. For we who are alive are always being given over to death for Jesus' sake, so that his life may be revealed in our mortal body. So then, death is at work in us, but life is at work in you. It is written: "I believed; therefore, I have spoken." With that same spirit of faith, we also believe and therefore speak, because we know that the one who raised the Lord Jesus from the dead will also raise us with Jesus and present us with you in his presence. All this is for your benefit, so that the grace that is reaching more and more people may cause thanksgiving to overflow to the glory of God. Therefore, we do not lose heart. Though outwardly, we are wasting away, yet inwardly we are renewed day by day. For our light and momentary troubles are achieving for us an eternal glory that far outweighs them all. We need to fix our eyes not on what is seen, but on what is unseen. For what is seen is temporary, but what is unseen is eternal" (2 Corinthians 4:7-18).

Well, that definitely put things into perspective. I guess it isn't all about me after all; is it God? Could all of this pain be for a reason? Alrighty then! I don't have to like what I'm going through. It won't help me heal any faster. Patience is a virtue, so they say (Whoever they are!). I'm just going to have to trust God for what He has to say about my situation. Without faith it is impossible to please Him. God help me have faith. I extend my faith that I will be healed in Jesus' Name!

What God was saying is, "This situation is not about you, it is about Me. I want all the Glory from this situation." I didn't feel like there was any glory; but, if He said He was going to get all the honor, glory, and praise from this situation then let it be. Let people see me working through the pain so that when I am making progress, they will see that, too.

The one thing I needed at this point was peace. I needed God to give me peace and comfort. I realized that it would take time to heal my foot. I had no choice but to wait and rest my body so that my foot would be healed properly. If I didn't do what the doctor said, then my foot would not heal properly, and I might reinjure my foot and have to go through the whole process again. My prayer was, "Lord, help me to get through this so that my foot can be healed, and I can go back to doing the activities that I could do before. I need some relief here."

I knew I had no choice but to surrender my situation to Him. It was totally out of my hands and control. I could not do anything about it. I had to accept that this was my life for right now and I needed to get over myself, so to speak, and not give in to the temptation to have a pity party. I would have to go through this time of healing. The life that I had known came to a complete halt. This would be a day-by-day process for me. My outcome for tomorrow will be based on how well I did today. My pain on any given day was directly related to the activity I did the day before. This included the amount of rest and care I did, such as elevating my leg, using ice, and taking all of my medications. Pain would always be a tell-tale sign of whether or not I was on track with my care.

There is a popular song on the radio with the lyrics, "What doesn't kill you makes you stronger" and that was the theme song for my life. I had to keep reminding myself that this is not my permanent situation and that I will laugh about this later. I held on to the scriptures, "Give thanks in all circumstances..." (1 Thessalonians 5:18). "Be merciful to me, O Lord, for I am frail; heal me, O Lord, for my bones are dismayed" (Psalm 6:2, BSB). All I can say is amen to that! When you are in constant pain you will go to any lengths to get relief but my attitude was always, "OK, God, I'm your vessel to show the world what you can do through me."

If you have ever seen metals being molded and shaped, you know they first have to be heated to make them pliable. Fire makes the metals workable and then extreme pressure makes the shape. We too become pliable when we are walking through the fire of life. Pressure will define and shape you. The definition of the word pressure is, continuous physical force exerted on or against an object by something in contact with it. When you constantly come in contact with pain, it changes you and you get to decide how.

When you surrender to the process of what God is doing in your life, it changes you for the better and you become stronger. A minister mentioned once that anointing only comes by crushing. You have to die to self to be reborn in the power of the spirit.

I took a steel drum symposium years ago where they talked about metallurgy, which is the study of metals. When you look at metal under a microscope before it is fired or what they call tempered, you can clearly see that the molecules are all over the place and not in any type of pattern at all. However, when the metal was observed after being fired or tempered, all the molecules were organized into rows and columns. When the metal was tempered it was very easy to bend. As Christians, our goal to be easily moldable into the image of Christ so we can reflect the teachings of Jesus. To do this, we cannot neglect the fire. We have to go through the heat which makes us more pliable. Heat isn't comfortable and in fact, it can be painful, but we to have to go through this process of refining and reshaping. Like the diamond that comes from coal, heat, and pressure make us beautiful and brilliant, reflecting God's glory. If you know that you are in the fire right now, consider yourself right now a diamond in the rough!

CHAPTER FOUR

Focus on the Finish

"Do you not know that in a race all the runners run, but only one gets the prize? Run in such a way as to get the prize. Everyone who competes in the games goes into strict training. They do it to get a crown that will not last, but we do it to get a crown that will last forever. Therefore, I do not run like someone running aimlessly; I do not fight like a boxer beating the air. No, I strike a blow to my body and make it my slave so that after I have preached to others, I myself will not be disqualified for the prize."

1 CORINTHIANS 9:24-27

After one of my surgeries, the nurse gave me papers that addressed my aftercare, what to do, or not do, and my instructions for taking my medicines. On the paper, it stated that the first three days would be to 1. Rest, 2. Take my medications, and 3. Eat. That was it. For me, there would be no problems meeting those goals. They were simple and small. I had to realize that was all I could handle at the time. When dealing with recovery, you have to be patient with yourself and do only what you can do for that day. It sounds easy enough but it's actually very difficult to change from a fast-paced routine, like most people are living in nowadays. Trying to do too many things will only frustrate you and cause the healing process to take longer. Give yourself permission to slow down. You are going to feel restless because something major has happened to your body. Your body is adjusting to the trauma of surgery. It feels different and awkward. Why can't you do the things that you are used to doing? Those feelings are natural. We have a society that tells us not to show any signs of weakness. This is not a realistic expectation. You are going to really have to watch your self-talk and not be hard on yourself. This is a temporary situation. Don't try to be a superhero! This is your time to chill and relax. I saw the following posted on TobyMac's social media account and I think it fits perfectly:

"Practice the pause.

When in doubt, pause.

When angry, pause.

When tired, pause.

When stressed, pause.

And when you pause...

Pray."

Speed is not important at this time. Make sure you are

never rushing or in a hurry. You will be learning how to be dependent on others, how to use medical equipment, and how to simply get from point A to point B. Make sure you are patient with others as well. They might not do things exactly the way you like or make your meals the way that you do. Eat the food and focus on being thankful that someone is taking care of you! Being grateful is an important part of your healing journey so chose each day to have a grateful heart.

We have to remember that when life throws us a curve, there are steps to getting through it. You may not enjoy all of the steps, but you have to know that God is working behind the scenes on your behalf. You don't have to have it all figured out before you take the next step. Just trust Him. "And we know that God works all things together for the good of those who love Him, who are called according to His purpose" (Romans 8:28, NASB). As time goes by, you will realize that this is just a season of time. You have to take the time to heal. There are no "skipping steps." In fact, if you try to push yourself too hard, you could digress and have problems with these injuries later in life.

How do you keep pacing yourself through the process? That is the whole premise of this book—don't rush it. Face each day as it comes. Don't worry about tomorrow. "That is why I tell you not to worry about everyday life—whether you have enough food and drink, or enough clothes to wear. Isn't life more than food, and your body more than clothing? Look at the birds. They don't plant or harvest or store food in barns, for your heavenly Father feeds them.

And aren't you far more valuable to him than they are? Can all your worries add a single moment to your life?" (Matthew 6:25-27, NLT). Life may not feel fair at times; however, worrying isn't going to help the healing process. Get rid of the negative thinking and set your mind in the right direction. This will uplift your spirit.

Remember, God knows where you are. He has not forgotten or abandoned you. "You have searched me, Lord, and you know me. You know when I sit and when I rise; you perceive my thoughts from afar. You discern my going out and my lying down; you are familiar with all my ways. Before a word is on my tongue you, Lord, know it completely" (Psalm 139:1-4). At this point, you just have to let go and let God do the rest. It is out of your hands. Do not be consumed by your problems. This too shall pass is an old saying; but true. This is only a season in time.

Don't Let Limitations Limit You

While you are learning to slow down all of your activities, you will start to see your limitations. This can be a very frustrating time. Before, you would get up from a chair and walk anywhere you wanted to go. There were no constraints before. However, now that you are recuperating from an injury you realize that everything is a struggle. How are you going to get from the chair into the bathroom with crutches? With a wheelchair? With a walker? Rugs will be your enemy. Rain, or anything wet while using crutches will be difficult. You have to be careful not to swing your legs when using crutches and keep your feet under your body. This sounds like a lot to think about; but I've learned from experience. Even though I'm talking about my physical limitations, the emotional struggle is real. Be aware that you will have a wide array of emotions that will come up. Have steps in place for you to deal with them. Talk to a friend, journal. Reflect on whether or not they are connected with people or your perspective of a situation. If you need to, call your pastor or get professional help.

One time, mom was going to get groceries. I thought I would tag along with her just to get out of the house. The grocery store would surely have an electrical cart available! Right? Wrong. They didn't. They were all being used. Great! Now what? There would be no problem using crutches while going all through the store looking for groceries. Right? Wrong. After an hour and a half hobbling all over the store on one foot looking for groceries, we were finished. Okay, I was finished. My legs were throbbing in pain. After that experience, my mom had permission to do the grocery shopping by herself and I was going to eat whatever she bought me.

Just remember, as frustrating as it is, everything takes so much longer to do. You cannot be in a hurry. From getting dressed to taking a bath, from maneuvering in bathrooms, to getting in and out of the car. No easy task. And the crème de la crème—going up a flight of steps. I would cringe inside at the thought. Ugh!

Another limitation for me was sitting through the service at church. We didn't have traditional pews, we had individual chairs so I would put one chair in front of me so I could elevate my foot. This position isn't comfortable for very long. All through the service, I would adjust my position to try to stay comfortable. I felt like a fidgety child constantly tossing around! The head usher would keep watching me and come over to ask if there was anything he could do to help. Bless his heart. He was always right there in seconds, but there wasn't anything that anybody could do. This was just my situation at that moment.

"...for I have learned to be content regardless of my circumstances" (Philippians 4:11, BSB).

Even though there are some things that you can't do, there is a lot that you can do. You can rest, relax, renew your mind, pace yourself, and most importantly surrender control.

"...in view of God's mercy, to offer your bodies as a living sacrifice, holy and pleasing to God—this is your true and proper worship" (Romans 12:1). I practiced an attitude of surrender and seeing myself as a living sacrifice for Him a lot while playing the piano for church services. I didn't feel like being up on the platform playing the piano while injured, on prescription medication and completely tired. But there I was—allowing God to use me as He saw fit. Not my will but Your will be done.

Look for Spiritual Parallels

There will be times in the process where you feel like you aren't certain if you have what it takes to get through this.

However, if you don't finish the process, and finish well, then how are you going to go to your next assignment? Now, it may seem strange to see the healing process as an "assignment," but it is. Even if you don't regain full physical use of your body, the process is to care for yourself, to support healing, and to keep your mind strong. My pastor is always saying, "First the natural and then the spiritual." We have to deal with the things that are going on in our lives in the natural because they are tied to the spiritual realm. For example, I had a couple of surgeries to straighten the big toe to have my foot aligned to bring balance to my body. As I thought about it and talked to God about it, I could see that in my spiritual walk, God was aligning me and adjusting me for my next assignment.

Going through these foot surgeries has truly given me knowledge and understanding about the process of healing and how God is healing me inside and out. Learning to see myself through God's eyes is humbling and amazing and causes me to rely on Him!

Another important part of the process, both spiritually and naturally, is stretching. Maybe you can't get on the floor and do full exercises, but you need to make sure you are moving your body as much as possible. You know the saying, "If you don't move it, you will lose it." Meaning, stretch and move whatever you can. You might not feel like it; but it is something that you have to do. Here's why: all of your soft tissue inside your body, known as fascia, is connected throughout your entire body. Any type of stretching is beneficial for your whole body, even the parts you may not be able to move because it's all connected. Again, I'm not suggesting hardcore workouts, just gentle stretching. NOTE: When you are going through healing, there are many days you won't feel like doing anything but sitting and being left alone. It's easy to let the hours slip by while you are in your comfy chair, but you have to make yourself move. Every hour, try to be intentional to get some sort of movement in. Make sure you get up and go eat at the dining room table, or somewhere besides where you have been sitting. Or, you could also do something simply like squeeze a small squishy ball for hand exercises. The spiritual implication here is that God is always stretching us. He is always increasing us beyond our limits. He wants to see us move out of our comfort zones because that is where we will see His glory.

Everything is Ordinary Until God Says It's Not

I was so excited to return to work after four months of non-weight bearing. I still had to maneuver with a boot when walking, and I had to wear a sneaker when driving, but the excitement was in the air none the less! On my way to work, there is a marquis sign that I would pass each day, that had some pretty funny sayings on it. On the day I was returning to work it read, "Crawling will still get you there." It made me chuckle when I saw it. It's like they knew I would be driving by! That line was such an encouragement to me. A couple of months later, there was another quote on the marquis, "Never turn your back on a charging turtle." I thought that was random and pretty funny, right?

Well, that night when I got home and went on social media, there on my feed was a video of a charging turtle! OK. What is going on here? Strangely, I started noticing turtles in my path all around me. At first, I didn't pay much attention to them. I grew up in Hartly, Delaware, which is way out in Amish country. There were a lot of turtles around. My brothers also trapped them and sold them to restaurants. No big deal! My pastor made a statement once, "Everything is ordinary until God says it's not." Wow! Why, but why, was I seeing tortoises everywhere? First, there were people with Green Turtle shirts on holding the door for me at a store. By the way, Green Turtle is a restaurant franchise. Then I would see a tortoise on the side of the road. Then there was a stuffed tortoise in the car in front of me at a red light. There was a turtle painted on a spare tire covering. Then there were the Ninja turtle shirts that people wore. Some of my friends would put a tortoise after their text message. One friend gave me a gift which was a tortoise with birthstones on it. And, how about the time I received a birthday card with a picture of a tortoise on a roller skate. No one knew that I was noticing a lot of tortoises, but it seemed I was being bombarded with them!

One Saturday afternoon, I prayed and asked God what this was all about. I spent all afternoon studying turtles. Some of my finding are as follows: The Logger Head sea turtle has an internal memory. They have a homing signal that takes them back to their birthplace, no matter how far out into the ocean they swim, no matter where the currents take them, they are always drawn back to their home and that's where they lay their own eggs. I too have been drawn back to my home in the natural. I moved away and returned, but even more so on a spiritual level. I think we all have an internal homing device that points the way back to God, our spiritual home. The Snapper Turtle is a feisty little fella and he will charge and bite down on anything that gets near him. Their jaw strength is amazing! Even without teeth they are powerful. They will snap, bite and cut with their beak. They have tremendous determination and resolve. The Giant tortoise grows to be 500 pounds and live to be 150-200 years old. How do they live so long? They have a slow metabolism. Slow and steady wins the race!

In 2016, the Teenage Mutant Ninja Turtles movie, "Out of the Shadows" was coming out. Well, after all these "turtle encounters" I had to see this movie. I'm pretty sure I was the only one to go see it with a notebook and pen in hand but I didn't want to miss a single insight. And yes, there were nuggets of truth that I wrote down as I watched this movie such as: People fear what they don't understand and by keeping unity in the team, you will have success. At the end of the movie, the Teenage Mutant Ninja Turtles found a potion that would turn them back into their normal self. They had a choice to make. They could live normal lives or stay the crime-fighting Ninja Turtles. They decided to throw the potion away. After which the Ninja Turtles stated, "What fun is that?"

In other words, they wanted to live an extraordinary life. They didn't want to be normal. They wanted to have a purpose and drive in their life. What am I saying? Your life is not over because you are dealing with pain. You may feel like a mutant version of yourself, but no matter what, if you take time and learn about how to care for your body, you can still do extraordinary things. You can be stronger in your mind and fly higher than you ever imagined. By being slow or slowing your life down, it doesn't make you less valued. You have to see beyond your limitations and see yourself through God's eyes. Even if you have to crawl. You have to keep moving forward. "Looking unto Jesus, the author and finisher of our faith..." (Hebrews 12:2, NKJV).

Your Mouth is Weapon

I mentioned earlier that I saw a video of a charging turtle one day on social media. It was quite interesting. You could see the passion in that little turtle even though he wasn't moving very quickly. But he kept walking—uh..charging—towards the person, continually opening and closing his mouth. As I watched, I felt like God was speaking to my heart and saying. "You may be crawling; however, your mouth is a weapon."

I propose to you, even though you are injured, physically, mentally, or emotionally, your mouth is still a weapon. You can speak life over your situation, and you can still pray. Pray not only for yourself and your present situation but pray for others as well. Speak what God says about you and your circumstances. "For though we walk in the flesh, we do not war according to the flesh. For the weapons of warfare are not carnal but mighty in God for pulling down strongholds, casting down arguments and every high thing that exalts itself against the knowledge of God. Bringing every thought into captivity to the obedience of Christ" (2 Corinthians 10:3-5, NKJV).

Another interesting thought about that charging turtle video is that the turtle never stopped moving forward even when the person moved back. He was not going to surrender until he hit his target. In the same way, do not surrender to your pain or let the pain win. Overcome your fears and charge forward into your destiny. No matter what, keep moving forward!

"Therefore...let us lay aside every weight...and let us run with endurance the race that is set before us" (Hebrews 12: 1, NKJV). Be sure footed. Be stable. "The steps of a good man are ordered by the Lord: and he delighteth in his way" (Psalm 37:23, KJV). We should be excited not because we are dealing with injuries but because each day is special. Each day is getting us closer to the fullness of our healing. Look at each day as an adventure!

Follow Your Doctor's Orders

After my first surgery, I substitute taught for a tap class. I was told to rest and not try to do the moves so I would pick a student to be the example in front of the class while I would call out the combinations and watch by the sidelines. No problem. At least that was my intention. As the class progressed, my feet got warm, the pain was gone, and so I let myself join in the routine. After class; however, my foot was throbbing in excruciating pain. This was 100% my fault. Did I listen to the doctor? No. Oops.

I had a follow up with my doctor the next day. What would I tell him? I only made it worse. Maybe he wouldn't see the swelling...Not. There would be no mention of the tap class that I taught. My lips were sealed. During the appointment, he unwrapped my foot and notices how it seems to be quite swollen. "The swelling should have gone down by now." He said. The guilt within me was overwhelming and I couldn't take it anymore. I had to confess what happened! The doctor was not happy. I was not happy. The dance teacher was not happy. This set me back. I had to be extra careful not to go back into activities until my foot was ready to go back to activities. Lesson learned!

You may want to be done with this problem and move on to the next step. But don't make the same mistake I did. Make sure that you are following your doctor's directions. Take the medication! You will not be able to function if you are in excruciating pain. Once you have started recuperating you will then notice that you have less pain and can take less medicine. Don't try to be a hero. Just take the medicine. I also want to interject a note here. When I was propping my leg up with a regular pillow, my ligaments above my knee became painful. I just happened to change from the regular pillow to a micro bead pillow for support under my knee. The pain went away. There is more "give" with the micro bead pillow. You will thank me for this later. Do not go against what has been said. Trust your doctor's orders to rest because in the long run, you are only hurting yourself. Don't try to push onto the next step before you are ready. You have to take baby steps. Be present where you are. Do what you can do right now. Progress will come. Keep progressing forward my friend. You will get there!

FOCUS ON THE FINISH

CHAPTER FIVE

The Mind Game

"No temptation has overtaken you except what is common to mankind. And God is faithful; he will not let you be tempted beyond what you can bear. But when you are tempted, he will also provide a way out so that you can endure it."

1 CORINTHIANS 10:13

I always enjoy games that help develop your brain and mental fitness such as crossword puzzles, Sudoku, Solitaire, Concentration to name a few. Doing brain exercises help your mind stay sharp and healthy. But first, you have to have the desire to develop your brain. If you don't see it as important, you won't do it. The same is true for our mental well-being. There is a saying that, "What you put in, is what comes out." If you always dwell on negativity, negativity will come out. If you dwell on positivity, positivity comes out. That's why it's so important for your focus to be on positive things. People have willed themselves to walk, when told they would never walk again. They visualized themselves doing the supernatural.

When I lived in Tulsa, Oklahoma, there was a season of my life that I was a personal assistant for someone who was involved in a car accident and suffering from a head injury. The car she and her husband were in lost control in the snowy mountains of Colorado. She instantly lost her husband. The car was still in array when burglars stole money, skis, etc. from the car. She literally was left for dead and when emergency workers finally found her in her car, she was unconscious. They transported her to the hospital not knowing who she was. A business card in her husband's wallet was the only information they had and they were able to contact her parents in another state. She was in a coma for six months. When she woke up, which is a miracle in and of itself, she told herself that she was going to walk again. And she did. She relayed the story to me and explained that it was a long hard struggle for her. But she did it. She eventually could walk with a cane. She was an amazing woman with an enlightening story to tell. Instead of letting the doctors tell her what she was going to do, she told her body what it was going to do. But she also did a lot of work to keep her mind in the right place and keep her spirit strong in spite of all the opposition.

How do you keep your mind strong? You have to protect it by guarding what you see and hear. You have to be careful about what you think about and the way you see yourself in your mind's eye. Be nice to yourself. The image that you have of yourself can either be an asset or liability. You need to see yourself as God sees you.

It's so important to keep a positive mindset. When you look at life, is the glass half full or half empty? Believe me, if you look for negativity, it will be found. The same is also true for the positive. Make sure that your mind is not so bombarded by negative vibes so that you can keep your thoughts pure. Be intentional about what you are thinking about and don't let your mind wander all over the place. Then you have to deal with traffic jams in your mind and it becomes easy to let your thoughts go in the wrong direction.

"Finally, brothers and sisters, whatever is true, whatever is noble, whatever is right, whatever is pure, whatever is lovely, whatever is admirable—if anything is excellent or praiseworthy—think about such things" (Philippians 4:8).

Human nature is often to think the worst in any situation, however, as believers, we are commanded to watch over our mind and tell our mind what it will think about. We have to be intentional to train our minds to think on good things. Judge each thought that comes to your mind and don't dwell on the negative!

"We demolish arguments and every pretension that sets itself up against the knowledge of God, and we take captive every thought to make it obedient to Christ" (2 Corinthians 10:5). It seems so simple you say! Yes, it is! We want to make it difficult. It has to be more than that. This is juvenile. "For my thoughts are not your thoughts, neither are your ways my ways," declares the Lord. As the heavens are higher than the earth so are my ways higher than your ways and my thoughts than your thoughts" (Isaiah 55:8–9). You have to accept what God says. It is that easy.

Choosing the right things to read and watch helps tremendously to keep yourself in the right place in your mind. Sometimes you will not want to read. Be intentional to watch positive, uplifting television to help you during this time. There is also an abundance of biblical messages/services that are available to watch on the internet. Even if the pastor is of a different denomination , you can learn something from a fresh perspective and you get to hear other people's stories, how they overcame their struggles and how they moved forward with the knowledge they gained from their experience.

Don't Take Yourself Too Seriously

"A cheerful heart is good medicine, but a crushed spirit dries up the bones" (Proverbs 17:22). Really, don't take yourself so seriously. Have a sense of humor. I grew up in a family with six children, so I had no choice but to have a great sense of humor! There was always laughter in the house. My father was the best storyteller—now, whether the stories were true or not is a different matter. But the stories were so funny. One time he told us a story about his two brothers and how one of his brothers charged at the other to punch him. The first brother held his hand out and stopped his brother's head while the second brother started swinging. But his arms were too short so he just stood there punching the air! We laughed and laughed as we pictured in our minds what he was saying. Be intentional to get around people who make you laugh. Sometimes just putting on a funny movie or TV show will help during this time. One of my personal favorites is the "I Love Lucy" show. She always cracked me up! I could watch those episodes all day and never get sick of them! One time my brother and I were watching the western movie, "Friendly Persuasion" starring Gary Cooper and Dorothy McGuire. It was about a Quaker family's life before the civil war and the struggles about the war versus their religious beliefs. It was very funny to watch and helped me to dwell on something other than my pain.

Movies are great entertainment for when your mobility is limited. Make a list of movies or television shows that you would like to watch while you are recuperating. Include funny, humorous and light drama. Your mind will not be able to concentrate on three-hour movies with a lot of different plots involved. This will be too much for you to take and it will frustrate you. Keep it simple and fun. At the same time, mix up your activities. Make sure that you don't watch television 24/7. Rest is also very important. Turn the television off. Turn the radio off. Turn the music off. Don't forget to add silence throughout your day. Silence is very powerful and beneficial for your mental wellbeing.

I have found that journaling is very therapeutic as well. Writing down your thoughts, how you feel, logging when you took your medicine, or who you talked to that day will help keep you organized and peaceful during the healing process as well. When you look back on the entries, some will make you laugh, some will make you cry. But, by documenting everything you will see how far you've come. You will start to see yourself changing mindsets about yourself, your life and your goals. You will learn who you really are. You will see that you are bigger than your problems and that your life is not just about you. You will see the big picture of the world and by doing your part you can make a difference. You will realize that this is not where you will be for the rest of your life. This is for a season only. Remember, don't focus on the problem, focus on the solution. This has happened to you, but it's not the end of your story, it's just a part of your story. What can you do to go forward in your life? What has to happen to get you from place A to place B? You are the only person who can answer those questions.

Don't identify yourself with your injuries. Identify yourself with who God says you are. What does God want for your life? Searching for answers will lead you to know God in a whole new light. "And without faith it is impossible to please God, because anyone who comes to him must believe that he exists and that he rewards those who earnestly seek him" (Hebrews 11: 6). You will learn that it's not the mountains that you will overcome. It will be yourself. You are the one limiting you. Life is a journey with its ups and downs.

I was going through Facebook one day and came across this quote, "Many people are actually afraid to heal because their entire identity is centered around the trauma they've experienced. They have no idea who they are outside of trauma and that unknown can be terrifying. They are only known for their injuries. How will they act when the trau-

ma or injuries are taken away? They fear the unknown."
"Therefore, do not worry about tomorrow, for tomorrow
will worry about itself. Each day has enough trouble of its
own" (Matthew 6:34).

Make sure that you do not put a label on yourself. It will
hinder your healing. Make sure that other people don't put
a label on you. Sometimes you will have to separate yourself from people who you thought were your friends. However, when an injury happens, they seem to disappear and
don't want to be around you. You need to surround yourself with people that are positive and want to help you go
forward. Do not hang around people that do not encourage
you or build you up. Life is too short to hang around people
that bring you down.

Also, don't have a victim mentality. Look what this person or that person did to me. Blaming others will not help
your situation. You think the grass is greener on the other side. If you were only over *there* your life would be different. Too many times that has not been the case. This is
called deception. You are only hurting yourself. It will move
you out of your destiny. This is why we really need to be on
guard with our thought life. You don't want to be alone because no one can stand to be around you. Remember, we
need people. No "Lone Rangers" allowed.

If you dwell in this mindset for very long, it will soon be
hard to get yourself out. You will become bitter, mad, and
angry at the world. You will shun the exact people that are
there to help you. Nothing anyone says to you will help you

because you have chosen to stay in the pity party. Have you been so angry that you make the situation worse? Have you ever heard of the phrase, "Don't bite the hand that feeds you"? This concept was printed by Edmund Burke in the 1700s. You need to be kind to the people who are taking care of you and your well-being.

While with my brother recuperating from one of the surgeries, I asked if I could have breakfast. He said that I could and while I was at it, make him breakfast. Now, normally that would be very funny. However, it was not funny at the time. I was thinking, "Really, dude." He did eventually make breakfast, which my body was very grateful for. Sometimes family rubs us the wrong way. Everyone knows I love humor. Just not while injured.

Don't be impatient for God to act on your behalf. "Wait passionately for God, don't leave the path. He'll give you your place in the sun ..." (Psalm 37:34, The Message). God will do what he says. "Keep your lives free...and be content with what you have, because God has said, "Never will I leave you; never will I forsake you" (Hebrews 13:5). He is there with you every step of the way.

Live Past Your Feelings

When it comes to moving forward in life, you have to understand your authority based on the word of God. Your success isn't based on how you feel; but on what God says. In the natural, you don't feel like being happy when your body is sitting in a chair and dealing with pain or depression. You don't feel like helping others when you need help yourself. The feeling of worthlessness comes into your mind and if you dwell on it, you will lose hope. You have to get yourself out of self-pity by not letting your thoughts dwell on your present situation. Even though you are injured, there are things you can do to help others. What could they be? For starters, simply talk to people. It doesn't even have to be in person. With today's technology, you can send hope and encouragement through texting and social media. You can pray for others. Look for ways to be a blessing to the people around you because God's system works on sowing and reaping. When you go out of your way to help others, you will be blessed in abundance in return. Not only that, it will help get you out of your funk and you will feel the depression or pity lifting off you.

One day when I was going to the grocery store, I was in a "funk" of a mood. I just felt disconnected. I had all of my groceries in my basket and I was heading for the check-out line. A thought came to me to pay for the person's groceries behind me, and I knew it was God speaking to my heart. I'm like "What?" There were several people in front of me; but, no one behind me. I was saying in my head, please don't let it be someone with a full cart. Lol! It was my turn to check out. As the cashier was scanning my groceries, a single mom with a small child got in line right behind me. She only had a few items in her basket. Hallelujah! I told the cashier that I wanted to pay for the young ladies' groceries. Both of them were stunned. The young mom started crying and hugged me and thanked me for the kindness.

What if I would have let the "funk" win that day? I would have missed the blessing of pouring into this young mother's life which ended up being a huge blessing to me.

Don't be afraid to surrender yourself to God to be used for His purposes. "For I am the Lord your God who takes hold of your right hand and says to you, do not fear; I will help you" (Isaiah 41:13). This is such a great picture just like your mom or dad holding your hand saying you're going to be all right. God is saying, "You're going to be all right." When we put His Word first place in our lives, that's how we become stronger in Him.

It's All Subject to Change

Remember, God saw all of your days before they ever started. He will use this in your life. Your life is not wasted. Your life is important. "The Lord will work out his plans for my life...Don't abandon me, for you made me" (Psalm 138:8, NLT). God has it all under control. He has your back. He is not going to leave you hanging. "being confident of this, that he who began a good work in you will carry it on to completion until the day of Christ Jesus" (Philippians 1:6). You will have to know that you know that He has your best interest at heart. Life might not go the way we planned; however, there is a plan. We just don't know about it. We are along for the ride. The mysteries of life. If we knew everything that would happen in our lifetime, we wouldn't be able to handle or grasp it. God knows this and gives us a piece of the puzzle one piece at a time. I read this marquis sign, "I am a piece of work in progress." This is true for everyone.

CHAPTER SIX

The One Thing That Changes Everything

"If my people, who are called by my name, will humble themselves and pray and seek my face and turn..., then I will hear from heaven, and I will forgive...and will heal their land."

2 CHRONICLES 7:14

Have you ever thought that you just didn't need anyone? That you could do things all by yourself? Maybe being independent is your strong suit. You've got this, right? Wrong! Sometimes people feel this way because they've leaned on others in the past and it didn't work out. They were hurt by people and made a vow not to need anyone ever again. Some people find themselves is so much pain that they are too ashamed and just want to be alone. Some people feel like others don't want to help so they think, "Why bother? I'm just going to be hurt again and then I will have more pain in my life." Have you ever felt like a doormat? People just walk all over you? Do you feel like you are stuck and your life isn't going to change? Is your pain weighing you down? Are you living in a dark cloud that will not lift?

You can't be an island to yourself. When you feel like you don't know what to do or where to turn, that's when it's time to pray. Believe me, there is power in prayer. I took a stress management class one time and I once heard someone say, "You have to believe in another power. We can't deal with issues by ourselves. We weren't built to. God sees your pain and wants to help you. He will not let you down." So many people give God a bad rap because they think He should have stopped situations from happening in the first place. They think, "If God loved me, I wouldn't be in this situation. So why did this happen to me?" I wish I had all the answers for you, but I don't. I can only tell you what I have experienced in my life and how I came to terms with my pain. Did I overcome pain completely? No. I still deal with it in my life. As I get older, my body needs more stretching so that my joints don't get stiff. As situations come from day to day interactions with people, conflicts will bring up emotions that I have to deal with, or they will cause turmoil in my body. Negative emotions can cause problems, to the point that they can lead to sicknesses and diseases in your body, if you don't deal with them.

From my personal experience, prayer is the one thing that changes everything. First, it changes your perspective on your pain and your situation. It can lift the weight off of your shoulders and remove the dark cloud over your emotion. It will impact your confidence so you can sit higher and walk taller knowing that pain is not going to control your life. Yes, you can live in confidence while still over-coming pain! It's a step-by-step, one day at a time kind of process. There is life to be lived while still dealing with pain in your life.

Some people are intimidated by prayer but prayer is sim-ply taking time out of your schedule to talk with God. When I was young and went to church, I saw people pray with great expression. They were loud and wailed, while waving a white handkerchief. Their eyes were closed and a lot of times they were on their knees. It was a little overwhelm-ing to me, but I assumed that this must be how we are to pray and the only way to pray. However, I've since learned that you can talk with God anywhere at any time and you don't have to be loud or cry or wave a white handkerchief while you do it. To me, prayer is just like carrying on a con-versation with a friend. It's that simple. Anyone can talk to Him. He's as close as the air you breathe. He is listening and He longs to hear from you.

"Then my enemies will turn back when I call for help. By this I will know that God is for me" (Psalm 56:9). God is for you and He will always be there for you. Pause for a moment and think about that. Say it out loud, "God is for me." Say it again. Let that truth sink down deeply into your heart. You have to know beyond a doubt that God will listen to you anytime 24/7. No matter what's on your heart, no matter how large or small the situation, God is waiting for you with open arms. Scripture says He never slumbers nor sleeps. He's not mad at you, He doesn't hold grudges. He doesn't get distracted. You have His total, 100% undivided attention. He wants to hear what you have to say. You don't have to go through any ritual or a formality to get God's attention. Cry out to Him. There are 305 instances of crying mentioned in the Bible. How does that relate to you? You're not the only one nor the first person that has cried out. I don't know about you, but, when I cry, tension is released. I feel so much better. My makeup looks a mess because I'm a horrible crier. However, I do feel better as if weight has lifted off of me. Why is that? I think it's because we have tried to deal with pain for so long by ourselves. We think that there are other ways to deal with it. We try to look for all the other options out there to relieve our pain. We go here. We go there. We pay money to go to this conference and that conference just to find answers. So much tension is built up. You have to release it. Humans are not built to hold on to tension. We have to let it go. Note here: I'm not going to sing the song, but I know you already are.

I want to continue with the thought of crying out. When I was little, I had five brothers and sisters, yet my mother would know which one was crying. Just by the sound. She never got it wrong either. She knew which one was crying. This is just like God. He knows which one is crying. He is waiting for you to acknowledge that you need help. He already knows that you need help. He knows your urgent cry, your voice. Your voice is very important. As my Pastor says, "You have authority in your voice." Going back to mom. I knew when she was calling just for me and not any other sister. I also knew when something happened and she's calling for me! The tone in her voice changed. The same is in your situation. When you've had enough, the white flags come out and you cry. Your tone changes. You release yourself to God. This is when things start to change. You know that has to be God because nothing you tried worked.

Sometimes the pain is so deep that it's almost like you're frozen and can't move. You're numb all over. You can't move. This is when you have to have other people pray for you. "We who are strong ought to bear with the failings of the weak and not to please ourselves" (Romans 15:1). "Carry each other's burdens, and in this way, you will fulfill the law of Christ" (Galatians 6:2). Ask for people to pray with you. Sometimes people will be praying for you and you don't even know it. This is the amazing thing about the Body of Christ. God will put your name in someone's thoughts so that they can pray for you. Each prayer is important. You don't know who is praying for you.

It was a Saturday night and I was working behind the scenes of a dance performance. After the show, I went home, took a shower and went to bed exhausted at 12:00 midnight. Around 4:00 a.m. I was awakened by a small noise that sounded like a mouse. I was listening intently to the sound in my head. My brain was trying to identify the sound. Through my grogginess, I was listening and thinking, "No, it can't be a mouse because the sound was not scampering. Mice scamper all over the place. This sound was moving in a straight line. "No, it can't be my mom and dad because they would have said, 'We're here.'" However, they wouldn't be in my trailer at 4:00 in the morning.

I'm listening keenly now. The sound is coming closer. My brain was waking up now. Someone is in the trailer. "It has to be the man next door," I thought. I don't want him to come into my bedroom. I looked around. There is nothing that I could use as a weapon. No books near me. No bat. No nothing. I put my glasses on and didn't know what to do. The next thing that happens, I see a light glowing on my hallway wall. Here he comes. Without hesitation, I jumped out of bed and became Xena: Warrior Princess. I started screaming, Xena's warrior cry. I went to the intruder and started jabbing him with my elbow. Between the warrior cry and saying, "In the Name of Jesus, you will get out of my house" I was pushing him out the door. The door by the way was deadbolted. So, I was jabbing him, screaming, and undoing the deadbolt while pushing him out of my trailer. All "In the Name of Jesus."

I was going to go run after him. However, since it was very early in the morning, I figured this was not a good idea. I went to the kitchen to see how he got in! There it was! A hole in the side door. He had rolled up my metal door half-way and walked right in unbeknown to me. Upon immediately calling the police department with my address, I also called my mom. Thank God she heard my telephone call. Note here: God always hears your telephone call. Just call Him up. Mom and dad were at my trailer before the police were. I showed them the hole. They were shocked.

When the police arrived, I showed them the hole in the door and described the intruder. They were asking about his appearance and did I know why he would want to break in. They also asked if anything was taken. I had no idea why he would want to break in and I've never seen him before. My purse was laying out in the open with money in it. Not touched. There was a brand-new Fender amp in the living room. They could have taken it; but, wouldn't have gotten far. It was very heavy. I did find out the following week that the trailer from the cul-de-sac directly behind me was a drug spot. That following week 17 people were arrested for drugs. The police officers had red flags on the area for months. My poor intruder thought he had broken into the drug trailer. All he was looking for was drugs. He found so much more than he bargained for. He messed with the wrong person that day!

The police were asking how he got out. I told him how I ran out of my bedroom like a bat out of hell with the Xena: Warrior Princess scream, and elbowed him, pushing him back toward the door. The two police officers were looking at each other shaking their heads in unbelief while I was recalling the story to them. One officer asked if the intruder had a gun. My response was, "I don't know." Both officers looked at each other and shook their heads. The officer asked if the intruder had a knife. My response was, "I don't know." Both officers looked at each other and shook their heads. I was wondering what they were thinking. They told me that a person is never to confront an intruder. Oops! I didn't know. However, now I know! Both officers stated that from their experience I should be a statistic right now. A dead person. This type of situation never has a good outcome. I stated my belief of Jesus keeping me safe. The report was filed and the officers left.

My brother showed up to fix the door that the intruder had entered. He had to unroll the door and secure it. After thanking him, he left. Mom and dad napped on the sofa and off to bed I went for a couple of hours. It was Sunday morning and we would be leaving for church soon. I got up-got dressed. My elbow hurt but didn't think anything of it. There was no time to look. We hurried on to church by 10:00 a.m. still groggy while talking about what happened earlier. This was crazy! So unheard of. What got into me that I thought I could take this intruder down?

There was a segment in the church service that the pastor asked for praise reports. I ran up because the adrenaline was flowing in my veins. I told the story and gave God all the glory and praise because he kept me alive. I should be dead right now; but, I'm not! People were shaking their heads as the story was unfolding. I, normally a quiet person, usually not a fighter, was elbowing an intruder out the deadbolted door as I was doing Xena: Warrior Princess cry. People started laughing, clapping and praising God for the miracle of safety.

After church, a gentleman came up to me and said, "Now I'm going to tell you the rest of the story." I said, "What story"? He answered, "Your story." He started telling me that God woke him up at 4:00 a.m. and said that someone was in need of prayer. He felt that this was urgent. God told him to pray and blow the shofar outside. His wife thought he was crazy. He thought he was crazy; but, he did it anyway. He thought, "What are the neighbors going to think"? He did it anyway. He told me that he did that from 4:00 to 4:30 a.m. He felt a release at 4:30 a.m. He felt that he had accomplished his task. He had no idea what it was for or who it was for. He was just obedient to what he felt God was telling him to do.

He was beside himself when he heard me testifying about the intruder and the time that this took place. He was so grateful that God used him to change this situation around. I was grateful that he was obedient even though it seemed inconvenient and crazy at the time. He saved a life. He saved my life. I thanked him for his obedience. "Greater love has no one than this: to lay down one's life for one's friends" (John 15:13). My friend didn't think of his inconvenience but did this out of love. Thank you, Jesus that there are people listening to His small still voice and taking action.

Obviously thinking about this now, how did I get this guy out of my door? It would not have happened on my natural strength. I'm not that good. Supernatural strength had come on me and it felt like I was in another zone. I just did what came to me without thinking of consequences. I was not even thinking about how he might hurt me or if other people were with him. I do remember thinking, "If I'm going down, he's going down with me. I was not going to give up without a fight." I definitely went into a physical battle, knowing that my weapons are not carnal but mighty in God for the pulling down strongholds. In this situation, for the pushing out of an intruder. This is Juanita's version.

My mom would keep asking me about the door. "Surely you heard the door being rolled up. What woke you up"? I didn't know what woke me up. There were no loud noises of any sort. The footsteps are the first thing that was heard upon waking up. In hindsight, I really feel that God woke me up. My spirit heard the shofar going off by my friend which was alerting me of danger. This is the only explanation that I have. I know this sounds like a farce; however, it happened and is documented by police reports as well as pictures of my elbow.

Just as I went into a physical confrontation with my intruder pushing him out of my house while hitting his back with my elbow, you might have to face emotional intruders and kick them out of your house. These intruders will stay as long as you don't confront them. They will take up house and live all around your family. You will have to go into battle and get them out. It won't be all of them at once; but, when God reveals an emotional intruder to you, make hast and get it out. The faster that you do this, the better. These strongholds have got to go. Don't entertain them with your thoughts. For you to move forward in your progress of relieving pain these emotions have to be stripped from your life. These emotions may not easily go. You have to scream out to God. You might have to do a prophetic demonstration and literally open your door and push them out the door. Take them by surprise so that they don't know what hit them. You have to tell them that they are not welcome in your house anymore.

"Truly I tell you, if anyone says to this mountain, 'Go,

throw yourself into the sea,' and does not doubt in their heart but believes that what they say will happen, it will be done for them" (Mark 11:23). These emotional intruders are strongholds. However, they can and will be moved. Enough is enough. Command them to go and don't make room for them anymore. Speak to them and demand that they leave your premises.

What are some emotional intruders: hate, fear, shame, depression, doubt, guilt, etc. There are a whole lot of them. They rob your spirit and soul of happiness, joy and all of the other fruits of the spirit. As the small voice brings an intruder to the surface of your spirit, deal with it. Be quick to rid yourself of it. Each emotional intruder that you get rid of is a step closer to your healing. You will feel lighter and happier. You could also have not realized that it was affecting your life or showing up as pain in your body. Every step that you take is a step of progress.

I took a long time on the above story. Why? Because I want you to know that if God did that for me, He will do that for you. I'm human, just like you are. Do I have any trauma from this situation? No. My elbow did swell up to the size of a tennis ball and was black and blue. Literally, I had tennis elbow! Lol! I realize that it could have had a different ending. However, I thank God that there was someone that took the time to do an unselfish act. Even though it seemed crazy to him at the time, it was for a purpose. We won't have all the answers–just a piece of the puzzle.

When I think of someone's name coming to my thoughts.

I pray for them. If I'm dreaming and see a situation with a person involved, I pray. When I hear an ambulance, see fire trucks, or see police cars with sirens, I pray. Why? Because someone did that for me and I want to pay it forward for someone else. I want to be that person that changes situations for the better. We are all put on earth for a purpose. I start one prayer at a time. I know prayer works.

We have to tell our testimonies to help other people. For them to realize God is not a respecter of persons. That what He did for me He will do for you. You just have to pray. There is no problem too great that He can't help. There is no person so far gone that He can't reach. You have to look up to God and just say, "Help." He wants to help you through your life. You will get to know Him at a deeper level through the pain that you experience. This doesn't make sense in the natural, but He wants you to help others by what you have gone through. The more things that you have gone through, the more people you can help. Everyone has different experiences and can help different people. I've never gone through a divorce, so I can't help people through their pain. I can help people that have had surgeries and have to recuperate from them. I've had loss in my family and can comfort others in that situation.

You will get a level of authority over things that you have been healed from. You have become an expert on how you got rid of things in your life. An example would be people that have become sick of their body, and the way it looks goes on a search for a program that will help them with their weight. They find a program and put the plan into practice. They lose a lot of weight. People start noticing that they are losing weight and want to know what they did to lose the weight. They start sharing with others what they had to do to get results. They are giving their testimony of what happened to them. The message is conveyed that you can lose weight also.

By telling people your testimony, you are giving people hope that they can be delivered also. You are telling your story. Your story has power. So powerful that you are telling people they can overcome their obstacles. They can go on with their life. We as people have to keep our hope alive. What are your dreams? Maybe you have let your dreams go because you held on to them too long, and you felt that they won't come to past now. So, you think!

"And the God of all grace, who called you to His eternal glory in Christ, after you have suffered a little while, will Himself restore you and make you strong, firm and steadfast" (1 Peter 5:10). "But those who hope in the Lord will renew their strength. They will soar on wings like eagles; they will run and not grow weary, they will walk and not be faint" (Isaiah 40:31). "The Lord delights in those who fear Him, who put their hope in his unfailing love"(Psalm 147:11). "Now faith is confidence in what we hope for and assurance about what we do not see" (Hebrews 11:1). There is a lot of scripture on hope. You have to hope for something. There is more to life than what you are going through. Hope for a better life. Let your mind dream again.

As kids, we always were daydreaming. Okay, okay, as a

kid, I was *always* daydreaming. I was always thinking of the future, and exploring my interests, curious about what I could do as a kid. Years ago as an adult, my church was doing a study on the book, "The Path," by Laurie Beth Jones. One of the exercises we had to do to help discover our strengths was to write down a list of all the things we enjoyed doing as a child. The scenario was to make believe that you would be paid $100.00 for each activity. The next week, each person stated how much money they would have received and I would have received thousands!

The point in this exercise is that your passions were being developed as a child. And it seems that when we grow older, we forget our passions, our dreams. I want you to encourage you to explore what your passions were as a child and write them down to help you begin to hope again. It doesn't have to be a long list. Let's start with one thing that you see yourself doing and start putting hope into. What have you always dreamed of doing? Begin doing something daily that will get you one step closer to your dream. If you want to limit yourself, the sky is the limit. However, God is a big God and there are no limitations. Let yourself dream again. Let hope rise up in your soul.

"Faith comes by hearing the message and the message is heard through the word about Christ" (Romans 10:17). As you hear what God says about you, you will become stronger. You will know that it's not your strength but God's strength. Music is a great motivator. Listening to the lyrics over a beautiful chord progression gets me every time. Think of songs that you love to hear over and over again.

Singing is a great way to lift your spirits. It takes you away from your present situation into the presence of God. You might start out quiet, but as you sing the words, there will be a boldness that comes over you. Before you know it, your spirit is refreshed and you feel like you can conquer the world. And you can. Because God's spirit is in you.

I had been dealing with a migraine on a particular Saturday, which carried over to Sunday. I'm a musician on the praise and worship team, so hearing a lot of sound around me isn't cool when you have a migraine. In the middle of worship, the song, "The King Is Among Us" was being sung. Suddenly the migraine went away. I was so relieved and excited that the pain was gone. I gave my testimony in front of the congregation to encourage others. Getting into God's presence is very powerful.

I'm going to leave this chapter with thoughts from Steve Harvey:

"Don't forget to pray, don't be ashamed to pray, and don't be too proud to pray. Prayer changes things. I don't care how dark things look to you. I don't care what anyone has said to you. Don't forget to pray. I don't care what the verdict is. I don't care what the haters say. Don't forget to pray, prayer changes things. If it wasn't for God, I wouldn't be standing here today. God saved me. Don't trip on my walk with God. God takes old hoodlums like me and turns them into Christians. I'm just a nobody, trying to tell everybody, about somebody that can save anybody." #Motivated on SteveHarvey.com.

CHAPTER SEVEN

Declaring, Meditating, and Listening

*"May these words of my mouth and this meditation
my heart be pleasing in your sight, Lord, my Rock
and my Redeemer."*

PSALM 19:14

What is declaring? According to Merriam-Webster, the word "declare" means to make known formally, officially, or explicitly publicly. It also means to make known as a determination. What are you making known as your determination? When a couple makes the announcement of their engagement, they are publicly declaring their love for one another. While keeping up with the royal family in England, they are always declaring an engagement, weddings, births. It's an exciting time because something is happening. Even the government of the United States of America is always declaring something. Remember the Declaration of Independence? It was the first step that the colonist took in telling the British government that they didn't want to be under their rule. The colonist made a formal document declaring what they wanted to become, even though the war for freedom lasted for years after that.

Why is declaring important? When you start declaring something, you get excited. You have the anticipation that something is going to happen. We see this in scripture as well. "The tongue has the power of life and death, and those who love it will eat its fruit" (Proverbs 18:21). "If, you declare with your mouth... For it is with your heart that you believe and are justified, and it is with your mouth that you profess your faith ..." (Romans 10:9-10, Parallel Bible).

I love what Shad Helmesetter said, "The brain simply believes what you tell it most. And what you tell it about you, it will create. It has no choice. If you tell yourself that you cannot, what can the only outcome be?"

When you declare positive truths about your future and declare what the outcome will be, it's like putting your foot down and telling yourself, "No more! I've had enough of this. It's going to stop." You have to start speaking about what you want to happen. It has to start with you, and it begins now. Make proclaiming statements that support the idea that you are coming out of this difficulty. You see the end. You are a valuable human being. You don't deserve to be stepped on. You are a caring individual. You are the only you that this world will know. You will use your talents to bring happiness to others. Start making a list of who you are, despite your pain.

It's so important to be intentional in focusing on the positive. Naturally, people tend to think the worst in any situation and go to the negative. If you catch yourself in a negative place, change what you are saying. Don't allow yourself to stay in a negative place.

As a music teacher, there are a lot of songs in my head. My friends see that as a positive as well as a negative. There is a song for everything! I just need to hear a few words and I'm off to another world with singing a song that pops into my head. Lol! One song that my class learned was "Think Positive." It had a catchy tune intertwined with rapping, uplifting lyrics. They loved singing it! This is an important reminder that even in pain, you can spread a message of love, light, and happiness to people. There is always someone you can encourage who is in a situation worse than yours.

How is this going to stop and turn a painful situation around? Again, the pain will take time to heal. I'm not suggesting that this will bring instantaneous healing. But this will help you make progress despite your pain. What are you going to do to make progress and move forward in your life? You are the game changer. No one else can change you. As you reflect on who you are and think about the person you want to become, just by having that awareness, you are changing.

Remember, you are stronger than you think. You do have the power to change things. As you develop your spiritual life and declare what God says about you, you will find the strength to overcome. When you become intentional to spend time with Him, I promise He will not disappoint!

"Now hope does not disappoint, because the love of God has been poured out in our hearts by the Holy Spirit who was given to us" (Romans 5:5, NKJV). God also wants to spend time with you and as you grow in your relationship with Him, you will see things change.

When I was in college, many moons ago, in a marketing class (yes marketing class) the Bible was a recommended reading source because of its positive and uplifting messages. The Bible was also recommended reading in English Literature classes. I would encourage you to get a Bible in a version that you understand and can relate to. There are so many programs on the internet to help you learn and grow in your faith. One way to learn more is to do a word study. Take a word and see what the Bible says about that word. See what dictionaries or commentaries say about the word. Keep a journal and write down any thoughts that come to mind as you are reflecting on the scriptures.

"Write down the revelation and make it plain on tablets so that a herald may run with it. For the revelation awaits an appointed time; it speaks of the end and will not prove false. Though it linger, wait for it; it will certainly come and will not delay" (Habakkuk 2:2-3).

Meditation

Another way to develop yourself spiritually is through meditation. In this day and age, we talk too much. We all keep so busy that we don't have time to listen. On top of that, when we are going through pain, our emotions are all over the place. Make yourself sit down in a quiet space away from the noise and away from life. Turn off the television, the radio, and your cell phone. I know this isn't easy. Oftentimes, my mind tends to be so busy that it is simply racing and hard to shut it off. I have to speak to myself and calm my mind. I declare, "I will meditate in thy precepts, and have respect unto thy ways. I will delight myself in thy statutes: I will not forget thy word" (Psalm 119:15-16, KJV). Once you are in a quiet place, just think about a scripture verse or truth from a devotional that hit your heart. Then simply listen from your heart. It's amazing what happens inside when we get still and quiet before Him!

Breathing Deep

Deep breaths are very calming to the mind and body. While you are meditating, praying, or just going about your day, take a few minutes to focus on your breathing. I like to put a diffuser on with some lavender essential oil. Lavender is known to calm the body as well. While you are breathing, close your eyes, and focus on your breaths. Don't take fast shallow breathes, take slow deep breaths. Count to three as you inhale and again as you exhale. Imagine peace going into your body as you inhale and the pain/problem or stress leaving as you exhale. This doesn't have to be for long periods of time. Start with a few minutes and see how long it takes you to be able to get in a calm zone. It's good to try to do this several times a day. Once you start doing calming exercises, you won't know what you did before you started doing them!

The Power of Music

Another way to bring peace into your life and connect with God is through music, whether it be inspirational, Christian, gospel, instrumental, etc. One time, I was given a plaque as a gift that was decorated with music motifs and simply says, "Music is the voice of the heart." This gift was so sweet and meant so much to me, not only because I am a music teacher, but the message rang true to my heart. Music is the one thing consistent in all cultures. Music is everywhere. Music impacts us on every level. Get into a beautiful quiet place, put on some music, close your eyes, and let it speak to your inner being.

Singing is also a great way to uplift yourself beyond your problems. It's an expression of you. It doesn't matter whether you sing on pitch or not. There is research that shows that humming ten minutes a day has a calming, relaxing effect on you. This explains why I was always yawning in vocal class in college! We would be warming up our voices with vocal exercises known as solfege exercises and people in the class would start yawning. I was hoping the professor didn't see me, but she always did. She explained one day that humming is calming and relaxes the jaw. This calming strategy is still current even though I learned this in 1980.

Once again, we see this in scripture: "Speaking to one another with psalms, hymns, and songs from the Spirit. Sing and make music from your heart to the Lord" (Ephesians 5:19). There's no right or wrong way to make a joyful noise.

You can even make up any melody you want. You can sing in your chair, couch, bed, in your car, or wherever you are!

One time, I was going to compose a song about my feelings during this phase of recovery in my life. I felt like I had hit rock bottom. I also knew that no one would buy a song that was entitled, "I Feel Like C***!" I was driving in my car one day (I do a lot of driving) and was feeling like my destiny and life was going nowhere. I felt like I had surgery after surgery and kept getting more pain and no relief. When you are so low, there's only one way to go: up. The car radio was on and the Whitney Houston song, "I Look to You" came on. It was from her comeback album (2009). I was overwhelmed with emotion, first because her crystal-clear voice was gone; but, also because the lyrics penetrated my soul. The song was like a last pitch of someone who was hurting very deeply. She had to look to someone other than herself, and so do we. Here are the lyrics to the song:

As I lay me down, Heaven hear me now, I'm lost without a cause After giving it my all

Winter storms have come and darkened my sun. After all that I've been through

Who on earth can I turn to, I look to you, I look to you, after all my strength is gone, in you I can be strong

I look to you, I look to you, Yeah And when melodies are gone. In you I hear a song

I look to you.

After losing my breath, there's no more fighting left, sinking to rise no more,

Searching for that open door.

And every road that I've taken, Led to my regret

And I don't know if I'm gonna make it. Nothing to do but lift my head.

I look to you. I look to you.

I could immediately relate to her and the words she was singing. She identified with my pain and my feeling that nothing was going my way and I needed help. The next day I went on a music website to pay for the sheet music to the song so I could learn it on the piano. This became my theme song. I had nothing left in me but to look to God, but that was all I needed.

Another way to build yourself up during difficult times is to listen to or read prophetic words that have been spoken over you. I have a prophetic file that has all my words through the years. Some are on old cassette tapes, and some on my cell phone. Some things I had forgotten about and as I read or listen to the words, my faith is renewed. I feel the excitement in my spirit. Even though I have a lot of these prophetic words transcribed from cassette tapes, sometimes when you're dealing with pain, you don't have the concentration or patience to read. Sometimes you just want to push play and listen to words that people have spoken about you and your future. If you do not have any prophetic words spoken over you, go to a trusted friend, pastor and ask them to pray for vision for your life. God is also a great source. You will learn a lot about yourself by listening to what He says about you. In that small still voice, He will bring thoughts to your mind. Do not throw these away. Keep them in your heart. Nothing is too big for God. If He gave it to you in the first place than He knows you can do it. God isn't in the business to make people fail. He is building you for success. Yes, success. Even when you don't believe in yourself. Even if you are hurting inside and no one knows what you are going through. God does and, He cares.

"Faith comes by hearing, and hearing by the word of God" (Romans 10:17, NKJV). As you listen, your strength from within will start to be awakened in you. Hope will start to arise in your heart. You have to have something that you hope for. "Now faith is confidence in what we hope for and assurance about what we do not see" (Hebrews 11:1). Without hope you will have no vision. You have to hope in something. Renew your dreams within you. Imagine yourself doing what you have always wanted to do. Just because you are dealing with pain doesn't mean that you can't dream.

Be Confident That He is Listening

How many times have you called someone on the phone and they didn't answer? Maybe it was a time when you needed someone to talk to right then and there. When there isn't anybody available to talk with me, I know that God is and He is my friend. "Draw near to God and He will draw near to you" (James 4:8, NKJV). God has already stated that if you take time to be with Him, He will come close to you.

Remember, when you do take time with Him, have your notebook and pen handy to write what you hear God saying to your heart. Start by thanking God for being there and taking the time to listen to you. Thank God that He has time for you. Reflect on what is in your spirit and write it down. Look for the nuggets that God will deposit into your spirit.

Always remember, by connecting with God through declaring, meditating, and listening, you are taking yourself out of your pain, both physical and emotional, and looking into your future. As you meditate and ponder things, ask yourself, where do I want to be in five or ten years? What you do today sets the course for tomorrow. Taking baby steps daily will get you where you want to go. There is nothing, there is no one who can hold you down unless you allow them to. You have full control of your life. Are you going to let this moment get the best of you or are you going to rise up and tell yourself the best is yet to come?

CHAPTER EIGHT

Waiting and Resting

*Patience is not about waiting, but the ability to keep
a good attitude while waiting.*

RECOVERYEXPERTS.COM

Have you ever seen a meme about waiting? It usually involves a skeleton or something dreadful. It implies that they have been waiting for so long that it is never going to happen. The person died while waiting. "I'm waiting for my wife to get in the car." It's a picture of a skeleton waiting in a car. "I'm waiting for my boyfriend to call me." There's a picture of a skeleton next to a cell phone. No one likes to wait for anything. We have drive-thru fast food. We have stores that have food already prepared. You just grab and go. I've been behind a car at a red light and as soon as it turns green, people start honking the horn! They didn't even give me a chance to take my foot off the brake! No one can be in that much of a hurry. But for whatever reason, everyone seems to be. We are an on-the-move society. There is no time for waiting. Go...Go...Go! There is only one speed, and that is fast! The faster we go, the more things we get done.

The definition of "wait" by Merriam-Webster: to stay in a place until an expected event happens, until someone arrives, until it is your turn to do something, etc.: to not do something until something else happens: to remain in a state in which you expect or hope that something will happen soon. As a people, we don't know how to wait. The notion of the faster we go or the busier we are, the more important we are. We have become so busy in our lives that when pain comes into our lives through situations, we feel that it has derailed our whole life. Our feathers are ruffled. Now what are we going to do? How could this be happening to me? What have I done for this to happen to me? We start taking things personally.

However, through this process, you will have to be patient with yourself. "But do not forget this one thing, dear friends: With the Lord a day is like a thousand years, and a thousand years are like a day" (2 Peter 3:8). Time is going to be your friend here. God didn't create everything in a day and problems will not go away in a day. "Let us not become weary in doing good, for at the proper time we will reap a harvest if we do not give up" (Galatians 6:9).

Healing takes time. You will learn a lot about yourself just by waiting. It is amazing. My sister died in 2017. My father died in 2018. Dealing with death is no easy task. Feelings of loss and getting through the fog in your mind is hard. By taking life one day at a time, you start getting pass the fog.

Slowly but surely. Things around you are moving while you are waiting.

When I went through one of my surgeries, there was a very popular song entitled, "While I'm Waiting," by John Waller. The lyrics are: I'm waiting, I'm waiting on You, Lord. And I am hopeful. I'm waiting on You Lord, though it is painful, but patiently, I will wait. I will move ahead, bold and confident. Taking every step, in obedience. While I'm waiting. I will serve You. While I'm waiting, I will worship. While I'm waiting, I will not faint. I'll be running the race even while I wait.

This song meant so much to me. This was the cry of my heart because, frankly, there was nothing else that could be done at that time. Here I am Lord. You will find me in a chair with my leg propped up. What do you want me to glean from You? I am relying totally on you. This was also a break from doing and being involved in so many things. This was a time of refreshing. A time for soaking in His presence. I didn't have to do anything for Him but spend time in His presence.

Sometimes while we are healing, we can get FOMO, or Fear Of Missing Out. Maybe you think that while you are waiting until your body heals, someone is going to take your place and do what you wanted to do or do what you feel you are called to do. The truth is, no one is going to take your gifts. Your gifts and talents are unique to only you. No one else can do what you are called to do. "A man's gift makes room for him and brings him before great men"

(Proverbs 18:16, AKJV).

You are going to have to watch your attitude during this phase because several things will come into your thought life. The first thing to watch out for is jealousy and the second thing to watch out for is anger. It's common to feel like you are being overlooked because of the pain that you are dealing with. You may have jealousy towards others because you think that they are not listening to you or that "they" look like "they" are all together and don't have to deal with what you are dealing with. You may be jealous of others because they can do things that you can't do right now—things you desperately want to do.

The frustration can present as anger. We usually take our feelings out on the people that we care about the most—our family. Why? Because we see them all the time. They know our strengths and our weaknesses. They know what buttons to push to get on your nerves. And they will push those buttons. However, we have to realize that when emotions are flying high, it is showing us something about ourselves. It could be that we have an unresolved issue from the past that we need to address. This is the time to deal with those issues.

If you don't deal with those issues, they will keep popping up in your life until you do deal with them.

While healing from injuries, and dealing with pain that comes with it, and waiting on God, He gave me a poem:

Rest in Me
Take the time to rest in Me
Let me hold you in My arms
Let me tell you that I love you
Let me show you that I care
Rest in Me

For while you rest in Me
I will give you strength
I will give you power
I will give you all that you ask

Trust in Me
Cast your cares into the sea
Let Me be your provider
Protector and friend

For while you trust in Me
I will give you wisdom
I will give you peace
I will give you all that you need

Believe in Me

For I have all the answers

I have all the world in My hands

For you are My child

You are so precious to Me

You are so sweet to Me

Please take the time and

Rest in Me.

I was so surprised at what came out of me as I journaled that day. Why would I be surprised that God would give me a poem while I'm in pain? I shouldn't have been. I used to write poems all the time, but I got too busy. All activity had to stop and I had to be forced to sit and rest to reconnect with my heart. And then, God downloaded a poem into my spirit. How sweet is that? It was like God could finally get me by myself and talk with me without any distractions. I have never forgotten that experience and continually strive to have quiet time with him amongst my active schedule. This is a priority for me and I hope you will make it a priority for you too!

While you are waiting, God will give you nuggets about your destiny and purpose. You will be able to look back and see how precious those times were when you were doing nothing but waiting. As boring as it seems, God downloads bits of information into your spirit that will catapult you into your next season. He is amazing like that! This will be the time that you will rise above average. People will see that you have changed because you have taken time to be with God. Your countenance will change. Your walk and stride will be more confident. You will no longer see yourself as defeated, but you will see yourself as God sees you.

The definition of "rest" according to Merriam-Webster: "a bodily state characterized by minimal functional and metabolic activities; freedom from activity or labor; a state of motionlessness or inactivity." I heard a sermon once about making rest as a lifestyle. We are actually called to live in rest. God created for six days. The seventh day He rested. If we are created in His image, we too need to take a day and rest from activity.

I'm not saying this is easy. In fact, this is very hard to do these days. There is so much activity all around us that it is very easy to get sucked up into going here and there and everywhere. Our brain goes into overload because of the stimulus all around us. It's like we are chasing an American Dream; however, it is at a great expense. Comparing your life to others is not the answer. That can become a vicious cycle and it's hard to stop the madness. Then we have to decide, are we going to do what we want to do, or are we going to do what God says to do? In life it is easy to keep doing what we want to do; however, this will not create the change we need to alter our current situation.

Change and growth don't happen overnight, which I have

already stated. It is a gradual, day by day process-one step at a time. You have to deal with your attitude one day at a time. But remember, you are in a temporary season. Just as we have stages in life, starting with the baby stage, there are stages that have to be taken to get yourself through this pain and recovery. You can make it easy or hard. It is your call. At some point you will look back on this circumstance in retrospect and say, "Boy, do I remember that situation that I went through. I don't know how I did it, but I did. It was all because of God's help that I came out of it." Let this be a stepping stone that will bring you into your next phase of life.

But also give yourself some grace. You are only human. You will make mistakes in your life. There has been no one perfect except one person and He was crucified! Sometimes we are our own worst enemy. It seems we can give patience to everyone else but ourselves! Give yourself a break because you can't do everything. If you try to, you are going to burn out. It's okay to not be able to do everything. It's okay to not be involved in a lot of activities. It's okay to feel tired. It's okay to show your emotions. And He said unto me, 'My grace is sufficient for thee: for My strength is made perfect in weakness. Most gladly therefore will I rather glory in my infirmities, that the power of Christ may rest upon me' (2 Corinthians 12:9, KJB). Where is your place of rest? For God yearns for a dwelling place. Let you be the place that God inhabits. For we need God's glory to rest upon us. "If you are insulted because of the name of Christ, you are bless-ed, for the Spirit of glory and of God rests on you" (1 Peter

4:14).

Make sure that you don't rush your healing and don't underestimate the power of rest. Healing is taking place while you are sitting and being still. Once we are at this place of rest, God can talk with us. He wants us to fellowship with Him. That's what we were created for. Think of a marriage relationship. Wouldn't it be awful to be married and not talk with your spouse? Or to not know what they like or what they hate? Or to not know their passion or what they desire to do with their life? God made us to commune with Him. "God is faithful, who has called you into fellowship with his Son, Jesus Christ our Lord" (1 Corinthians 1:9).

We have so much activity going on that we can't even hear what God is saying to us. However, when dealing with pain, we now are at a place to say, "What do you want God?" He says, "Be still, and know that I am God..." (Psalm 46:10). Make the most out of this time. Relish in the refreshing that God is giving you while you are healing from the pain. Get to know Him and what His word says about you. He is a loving God and wants the best for you. He wants to protect you while you seem vulnerable during this process. "He will cover you with his feathers, and under his wings you will find refuge; his faithfulness will be your shield and rampart" (Psalm 91:4). You will be taken care of during this time with God and with your family. It's like a father protecting his children. He won't let anything happen to them. He will be right there.

God wants to hear about everything you are thinking and

feeling during this time. Tell him about your frustrations and shortcomings. He knows about it already, but He wants to connect with you in a deep, personal way. "You have searched me, Lord, and you know me. You know when I sit and when I rise; you perceive my thoughts from afar. You discern my going out and my lying down; you are familiar with all my ways. Before a word is on my tongue you, Lord, know it completely. You hem me in behind and before, and you lay your hand upon me. Such knowledge is too wonderful for me, too lofty for me to attain" (Psalm 139:1-6).

The Importance of Self Care

During this time of waiting and resting, it is also important that you reflect on your own self-care. It becomes really like a checklist. Are you taking your medicine? Are you drinking your water? Are you getting enough sleep? I do know that when you are in pain, some of the first things that go is self-care. There may be times when you don't feel like eating or you feel that you are inconveniencing others by needing their help. We naturally try to take care of everyone else first and ourselves last. But even if you are injured and can't do a lot of activity, there are exercises you can do to help keep your strength up. If you are non-weight bearing, like I was, do stretching exercises using your hands. Touch your toes. Do side bends. Keep yourself actively stretching as much as you can.

Some things will be out of your control. When I was non-weight bearing, my blood pressure was very high. I was in the doctor's office when the nurse took my blood pressure and kept looking at me. I felt fine. Normally my blood pressure is low. That particular day it was through the roof. The nurse left my room to converse with the doctor.

During that time, my doctor wanted the school nurse to take my blood pressure every day. He wanted to keep track of it. I found out that pain elevates blood pressure. Also, because of inactivity for four months, I gained a lot of weight. I went from doing ballet three times a week and Zumba two times a week to nothing. I had to let my body weight go by realizing it was only for a season. The weight would go back down when activity would start up again. This was hard for me but, I had to let it go. And yes, I am singing that melody from "Frozen" right now. And, so are you! LOL!

You are responsible for what you can do and not what you can't do. For each person it will be something different. Taking care of you so that you can get healed is your focus right now. This does not mean that you are out of this race called life. No! It just means that while you are resting and waiting you are getting stronger. There's a song on the radio by Kelly Clarkson that states, "What doesn't kill you makes you stronger." This is really the truth! You might have been knocked down. Don't stay down. Get back up. Brush yourself off. And get back in the race. Life is too short and precious for you to stay down in defeat. There are also many things for you to do. Get ready. Get set. Go. And don't forget to rest!

CHAPTER NINE

The Power of Perseverance

"Not only so, but we also glory in our sufferings, because we know that suffering produces perseverance; perseverance, character; and character, hope. And hope does not put us to shame, because God's love has been poured out into our hearts through the Holy Spirit, who has been given to us."

ROMANS 5:3-5

According to Merriam-Webster dictionary, the definition of "perseverance" is: "continued effort to do or achieve something despite difficulties, failure, or opposition; steadfastness."

When going through pain, sometimes you just want to "throw in the towel" so to speak. There are times when you don't feel like doing anything and you can physically become lethargic. You're going to need some sort of motivation to get yourself out of the cycle of daily doing nothing. Start by seeing each day as a precious gift. This will help you to not waste the time that you've been given. Dig deep and find the strength to persevere because you have purpose and you can make a difference even in your current circumstances. "Therefore, do not worry about tomorrow, for tomorrow will worry about itself. Each day has enough trouble of its own" (Matthew 6:34).

If you think you are going to wait until you have no pain or trials in your life to do something, you will have lived your life doing nothing. I've heard the saying, "If you wait for the perfect time to have a baby, you won't have a baby." There is no perfect time to do anything. You have to make your own path in life and progress for tomorrow starts today. If you feel overwhelmed, break life down into the smallest steps possible. Think about what you can do right now that will help make your life better in the next minute. Yes, start with a minute. Then focus on the next two minutes. Maybe you take life in 15-minute increments for a little while. Start small and just think, what do I need to do in the next 15 minutes?

One time I saw a framed saying by Vivian Greene that read, "Life isn't about waiting for the storm to pass. It's about learning how to dance in the rain." This statement summarizes the premise of what this book is about. Don't wait for things to line up in your life before you do anything. A lot of times, you're going to have to do things while you're going through a storm. We've all heard the saying, "When life gives you lemons, make lemonade." Make your life count. Do something with what life has dealt you. I could easily say, "Oh, my hips hurt, my legs hurt I can't do anything. I can't stand up for long periods of time. I can't sit down for long periods of time. I'm up down up down!" Doctors have told me, "Stop dancing. You are reaching that age. Each dance you do could be your last dance." Do I listen to them? No, not at this time. Why? Because my body was made to move and movement makes me feel alive. There's a song that I love entitled, "Every Move I Make." It says, "Ev'ry move I make, I make in You. You make me move Jesus. Ev'ry breath I take I breathe in You. Ev'ry step I take I take in You. You are my way Jesus. Ev'ry breath I take I breathe in You." (Words and music by David Ruis) This is my prayer and this is my motivation. Jesus is my motivator to do what I do.

As a little girl, I always loved listening to the piano being played. I loved watching Liberace and Jo Ann Castle, on the Lawrence Welk Show tickling those ivories! I was so fascinated by how their hands just glided over the keys. As a young girl, whenever I was babysitting for someone who had a piano in the house, my hands were always experimenting on it. I loved it! Fast forward to when I was scheduling for a college semester, I noticed a beginner piano class open to all non-music students. My heart leapt with excitement! Could this be possible? Anyone can take the class? This was my opportunity—this class was mine! I started telling everybody that I was going to take a piano class. You wouldn't believe the feedback I got. "Well, you know you're too old." "You'll never be able to learn it." "You should have started when you were a kid." "Boys make better pianists than girls."

What? I was only 19. What could be so difficult? I couldn't understand the backlash over trying something new. Something that I have always wanted to do. Some of these people didn't play the piano anyway. How would they know how hard or easy the classes would be? It was only one semester. The cost was part of my tuition and went toward my college credits. I was thinking this through logically and trying not to let the negative comments get the best of me. To me, it was a no-brainer. I've never tried it. I wanted to try it. The opportunity is here. I'm going for it! I wasn't going to let the comments and beliefs of others determine my destiny. This was my education not theirs, my life not theirs. My choice not theirs. I made my decision and I also made the decision to not be upset or bitter at people. Maybe they had a bad experience with the piano. Who knows?

I could have just as easily said, "Oh well, I guess I can't do this. Why try?" But I didn't. The comments of others actually fueled the fire within me. Something rose up in my spirit that made me want to play the piano more than ever! I was going to show them and prove them wrong. This might not have been a good attitude to have; however, God used it anyway.

When I went to sign up for the class, it was already full. The registrar's office told me to talk to the professor. When I went and spoke with the professor, she stated that a lot of students will drop out of the class and suggested that I still come to the first class, so that's what I did. I went to the first day of class and sure enough someone didn't show up and I was moved into the open spot. I was focused and very studious because this was another passion from my child-hood that was coming to past, a dream being fulfilled. If the professor said to practice one hour daily, I would practice two hours. I was like a sponge soaking up everything the professor was saying. As time passed, more and more students were dropping out until I was the only one taking the class. She told me to meet her in her office the following week. What? I was going to be taking private piano classes one-on-one with the professor. Wow! What an honor and privilege.

After the semester ended, I asked the professor if I could continue with piano lessons. She stated that it was only for one semester for non-music majors. I would attend monthly music seminars and do what I could to keep learning. The professor came up to me at one of the events and said that she changed her mind. As long as she was faculty, I would be able to take piano lessons with her. I was on cloud nine and so thrilled! What an unfolding of emotions.

To this day, I remember her rigorous teaching methods. I remember her expertise and her passion that she encouraged me with. To look back and realize that I have been playing the piano now for over 40 years is truly astonishing. To think that if I had listened to people's negative comments, I would have never known the enjoyment of playing the piano. I play not only for my personal enjoyment but, for church, weddings, students, etc. God gets all the glory for giving me this opportunity.

To think, I was just one thought away from giving it all

up. I want to encourage you, don't let your thoughts or the thoughts of others hold you back. Press on and get motivated to improve your life for the better. Sometimes you will feel emotional pain from people who don't even know why they say negative things to you. It's usually because of their emotional pain or experiences that they give others wrong advice. Don't let it stop you! Look beyond the natural and see yourself as God sees you. See yourself rising above your circumstances.

When I became 39 years old, I realized I wanted to do something on my "Bucket List." I wanted to do something for me. So, what did I do to change? I had always wanted to take a dance class, and since I wasn't getting any younger, I called around and visited different dance studios in the area. I chose one that was not too far out of my way and that I felt very comfortable with. In my first dance class I noticed I was the oldest and the biggest person taking the class. That could have intimidated me; however, I chose to focus on the fact that I was taking a dance class! That was a huge win for me and I love, love, loved it. This was my form of exercise and it still is after 21 years. I may be one of the oldest, but I'm like the studio mom to all the kids who are also taking dance. Was I good at first? No. But, I kept going back for more. There were four classes that I took that first summer: social dances, jazz/tap, and two ballet classes. Was it easy? No. Was I learning something that I always wanted to do? Yes!

It wasn't all easy though. Very often, the next day after class, my back would be in excruciating pain. But I kept going. I learned by consistently going to class, my body felt better and over time, my back was having less pain. I was getting stronger all while learning a dance form that I've always loved watching. This was a win-win situation for me. I took action on something that I always wanted to do and I have never regretted doing this! You won't regret taking action on your dreams either, even in the midst of pain.

What motivated me to do this, to put action to my thoughts? For me it was my life's timetable. I didn't want to regret not doing something as I looked back on my life. At 39 years of age, my body wasn't getting any younger. I didn't know if it was too late for me or not. I wasn't sure if my body could do the moves. I wondered if I was going to look stupid or silly and I'm sure I did, but what kept me going was perseverance and sheer determination. I did not give up or quit. I kept showing up for classes. My legs would feel like jelly. I would get cramps in my legs in the middle of the night, or sometimes during the day. These symptoms were not going to stop me from going to class. I had a made-up mind. People thought I was crazy because I would be in classes with much younger kids. I'm talking 5 and 6 years old because I had never taken dance classes before. I stood out like a sore thumb. I didn't care. Sometimes I would ask for their help in showing me the moves. They liked that, of course. Everyone knew who Ms. Nita was— the adult taking ballet classes with the young kids. But this never deterred me from the passion that was inside of me.

"Is not my word like fire,' declares the Lord, 'and like

a hammer that breaks a rock in pieces'" (Jeremiah 23:29). Remember, your life is being chiseled into pieces, or baby steps if you will. A lot of times we can't handle the Big picture. This is why God is so great. He breaks it down into smaller pieces for us. As you take steps in front of what motivates you, you will begin to get clarity in your life.

You have to ask yourself the question, "What motivates me?" What passions do I have inside of me? Everyone has greatness inside of them. Everyone has talents and skills that once you begin to use not only brings you great joy but others as well. You will have to look within yourself and begin to pursue them. The definition of pursue is to follow (someone or something) in order to catch or attack them, chase, to follow close upon, go with or attend. Don't wait for the opportunity of a lifetime to come your way. You have to go after them. When opportunities do come across your path, you do have a choice to take hold of it or let it pass by. Timing is everything.

When the timing is right and you feel to go after an opportunity, do it with energy and enthusiasm. When you have passion, you don't let anything in your way. You keep the mindset on the end result. You don't think about the negative; you have people in your inner circle that are positive and have the same drive as you do. This attitude is what I am talking about concerning perseverance. You are so set on a goal that you do what has to be done to obtain the goal. "But I discipline my body and keep it under control..." (1 Corinthians 9:27, ESV). You are so focused on the goal that you are not bothered by inconveniences. This doesn't mean that you won't have problems come to you. It means you work through the problems and keep going.

I'll give you an example of the Olympian athlete. They are focused on their event: nothing more, nothing less. They watch what they eat, how they approach their workouts, how much sleep they get, etc. They are consumed with the outcome of their goal: to be an Olympian. When they get injured, while it is a setback, they are still focused on their goal. No one can deter them! They see themselves winning a gold medal in the Olympics and they won't stop until it happens. This is what it means to have perseverance.

They have to sacrifice their time, energy and family life to accomplish their goal. It is a hardship. It's not easy. It's an all-consuming goal; however, they want to accomplish it. They want it so bad they can see the medal in their hands, they see it in their hearts and sense the victory. It is theirs for the taking. Yes, it is a sweet victory, but the medal represents so much more. It represents the years that they had to sacrifice to make it happen. The ups and downs. The highs and the lows. They had to battle to the point of exhaustion.

They know first-hand the journey that they had to take to accomplish this feat. So even when they see the medal, the athlete realizes what it represents: the hardships, the sacrifice. A bystander doesn't see the years that it took to accomplish this. They only see the glory part. The exciting part! The cheering from the crowds. No one knows what kind of battles that had to take place to get the athlete the results. This is why you see so many athletes crying when they have won medals. Their path has been an emotional rollercoaster. They have finished the race and it was all worth it!

CHAPTER TEN

You Are Not Alone

"Be strong and courageous. Do not be afraid or terrified because of them, for the Lord your God goes with you; he will never leave you nor forsake you."

DEUTERONOMY 31:6

When you face an injury or any problem for that matter, it's natural to think that you are alone in your suffering and that you are the only person who has ever gone through something like this. It is only by talking with other people that you find out that this is not the case. "That which has been is what will be, that which is done is what will be done, and there is nothing new under the sun" (Ecclesiastes 1:9, NKJV). While going through many of my injuries, one at a time, I have become sensitive to others around me in similar situations. I have gained awareness of the people around me who are on crutches, in wheelchairs, with medical boots, and those using canes or walkers.

I always felt like I was in a different category of people:

those injured and recuperating from surgery. These people were my "tribe." Any time I was out and about and would see someone who was injured, it was just natural for me to start up a conversation. I would ask them what happened and when. I would share my story and ask them about their recovery plan and we would start encouraging each other that this difficulty is just for a season, and life would be back to normal in no time. I would strike up a conversation with people anywhere, sometimes on the streets while running errands, other times in the waiting room of a doctor's office. Connecting with people who are facing a similar situation brings comfort, strength, and insight and empowers you for the days ahead. It's important to have a network of people you can trust to support you on your journey.

See Your Doctors as Partners

Another group of people who I learned to trust were my doctors. I do not have a medical degree and to be honest, you would not want me to be practicing medicine. I know my strengths and weaknesses and I knew I need to listen to what the doctors said and follow their directions. If the doctor told me not to walk on my cast, I didn't walk on my cast. I knew that by following their instructions, I would get healed faster. It was a simple truth that made sense to me. Sometimes, however, I would follow their advice 100% and still have problems. But I still had to trust my doctors and go back to them and see if we could solve the problem. My doctors were my partners. We had the same goal: to get my body on the road to recovery so that I could go about with my normal activities. We definitely had a great working relationship and they were amazing, patient, kind, and honest.

Relying on Family

Another group of people I had to rely on was, of course, my family. As crazy as they are, family is family and they were needed. Every family has their strengths and challenges as a whole and we have to focus on drawing from their strengths at this time. My family has a great sense of humor and teased each other a lot. You cannot be thin skinned and survive in this family! My family's sense of humor is what got me laughing at my situation and laughing at myself. The Bible does talk about humor in Proverbs 17:22, "A merry heart does good, like medicine, but a broken spirit dries the bones." The choice was mine. Will I laugh about my situation or will I become a depressed and broken spirit? I chose to laugh because laughter helps take the sting out!

After my first surgery, I arrived at my mom's house for recovery. I was so careful getting out of the car. I got my crutches and started slowly making my way to the front door. I arrived at the front steps and just stopped and starred at them. Then I just started laughing so hard! I had no idea how to go up the stairs on my crutches! Hello...how was I going to get up the steps and into the house. My mom was right behind me and when she realized what was happening, she started laughing and laughing. Here we both are laughing hysterically, and she starts trying to help me up the stairs, pushing my backside and giving me a wedgie in the process! She was not helping which made it all even funnier! The neighbors came out and they started laughing at the scene and they all helped me maneuver into the house. We did get into the house. What a workout! I realized at that moment that steps were my enemy. At least going up. Going down was easy, as long as there was a banister. Of course, there was no banister at mom's house. Before going anywhere, I would always ask if there were steps and a banister! In case you are wondering, the best practice for crutches is to not use crutches going up steps but to sit on your butt and scoot up one step at a time. And now you know! You're welcome!

After several surgeries, my brother offered to let me recover at his house. He had a ramp which was so much easier to navigate than steps. I was using a walker with wheels at this particular time and I would put one knee on the seat and walk using the other leg. My walker had a seat with a storage compartment hidden under it. All kinds of stuff fit in that compartment: tissue box, cell phone, petroleum jelly, lipstick, water, word finds, sudoku puzzles, etc. Lots of stuff. I felt independent and was glad I didn't have to rely on family to get things for me because I had most of what I needed with me at all times.

At night, when everyone was laying down and trying to go to sleep, I, of course, was wide awake because of my medication. The medication was supposed to make you drowsy, but not me! It seemed to have the opposite effect and I found myself wide awake many nights. My younger brother was visiting at the time. At nighttime he slept on the couch because there was not a guest bedroom and my other brother slept in a lazy boy chair because he was having trouble with his back. I was in a Lazy Boy chair with my foot propped up on some pillows. The nights went very slow for me. I couldn't sleep, as usual, and would keep going in and out of the storage compartment in my walker finding things to do. Every time I opened and closed the lid, it would make a piercing squeaky noise. It was so bad... how bad was it? The walker became known as, "Squeaky." Every time I would need something—squeak up, squeak down. I needed something else—squeak up, squeak down. I was proud of myself for being independent and I was not payng attention to the noise which was certainly affecting my brothers trying to sleep in the same room as me. Until my younger brother, Gerald, with both eyes still closed gruffly said, "If you open Squeaky up one more time, I'm going to throw it outside!" Oops! I guess I don't need anything else! I can't tell the story as well as my brothers because they have the noise of Squeaky down to perfection. Of course, they add their drama flair to the story. Whenever we get together, this story always surfaces.

Relying on Friends

Another group of people that I had to rely on was the worship team at church. I did my best to keep my commitment to play the piano during my recovery, even though I was still non-weight bearing. Thank God the worship team was not moved by my situation or the look on my face. Many times, I would be playing the piano with pain and head-aches and my face would definitely show it. Sometimes I would be at rehearsal and could feel the medication wear-ing off. I would tell them, "You have ten minutes and then I'm done." My body knew when I had enough and I could count on my friends to support me. I knew they had my back. They prayed for me. They helped me down the steps. Remember, down was the easy part!

One time I was reading the worship group text thread and someone sent a message that said, "Hey, do you guys know that Satan and Santa share the same letters?" Obviously, the medication took over because that someone was me! I don't even know where this thought came from. One of the singers, Sharese, whom I've known for many years, imme-diately told me, "Put your cell phone down. Don't get on Facebook. Don't call or talk with anyone. You need to get off all social media and go take a nap!" She was right and I'm glad she loved me enough to tell me.

When you are going through rough situations, you need friends who will be real with you. Friends who have your back and will tell you that you are in left field and reel you back in. We all need friends who will encourage us and make us laugh, friends who will give you positive feedback and love. Thank you for the reality check, Sharese! Also, thank you worship team for sticking with me even when my attitude was not the best. I appreciate your love and un-derstanding during the hard times.

Getting Through the Wilderness

With all my activity coming to a halt, I felt like I was in a wilderness experience: nothing happening in my life, God didn't seem to be talking to me, I had feelings of being alone. Maybe you've felt that way too. During this time, I felt like I had nothing to give anyone because my own situation seemed so overwhelming. I want to propose to you that we have to go through the wilderness experience to get our promised land. There seems to always be a valley before you get to the mountain top. In the natural, if you are in a desert, your brain starts to see things that aren't there. You begin to get delusional.

Jesus went through a wilderness experience. He was tempted by Satan who took Jesus up to the mountain. While there, Satan was twisting scripture trying to make Jesus submit to him. Jesus would quote scripture back to him. This is a powerful example that when we are at our weakest point, we have to quote what is written in the Bible instead of our interpretation. Tests will come. We can't stay in the wilderness. We have to pull ourselves up to the mountain and see ourselves the way Christ sees us. We have to keep our eyes on the mountain of God. "The voice of the Lord shakes the desert" (Psalm 29:8).

Do you remember when Moses went up to the mountain? He went up and beheld God. He talked with God and God gave him the Ten Commandments. When you go up to the top of a mountain, you can see everything around you with a new perspective. The view from the mountain is beautiful. It's awesome and awe-inspiring. You're not bothered by anyone or anything. You want to hold that moment and capture the picture in your mind. This is how God wants us to be. He wants us to see the big picture and how we fit into the big picture. He wants to take us up to the high places in Him. God is not a tormentor. He is your loving Heavenly Father and He wants the best for you.

When you are in the wilderness, you will find your voice. The wilderness hones your faith and helps you become grounded in truth. During this time, go to the Bible and see what God says about your situation. Let God's word give you hope, vision, and clarity.

"I waited patiently for the Lord; He turned to me, and heard my cry. He lifted me up out of the slimy pit, out of the mud and mire; He set my feet on a rock, and gave me a firm place to stand. He put a new song in my mouth, a hymn of praise to our God. Many will see and fear the Lord and put their trust in Him" (Psalm 40:1-3).

I realize that the wilderness is not a fun place to go; however, it is a necessary passage that everyone has to go through. You have to know that Satan, the accuser of the brethren, wants you to lose your voice and feel discouraged during this phase of the healing process. He wants you to feel like you are alone and that no one cares about what you are going through. He wants you to have your pity party. He also knows that you have a purpose while living on this earth and his goal is to stop you from fulfilling it! If God is for you, who can be against you? God is on your side, but you will have to battle for your vision. No one is going to hand it to you on a silver platter.

Divine Encounters Are Coming

Have you ever seen the movie, "Close Encounters of The Third Kind"? In this movie, people had encountered aliens and you knew it because they were either sunburned on a part of their body, or they knew a particular melody from the meeting. Many people in different countries had seen the UFOs. The research teams were trying to keep the people away from this designated mountain. Friends and families of these people didn't understand why they were becoming so obsessed with going to this particular mountain. Their families thought they were crazy. These people had definitely seen something. They left everything behind and felt drawn to this mountain. Even when a lot of people got close to the mountain, there were obstacles put in their way by the research teams. This project was a secret. They were told to turn around and go back home. They were not wanted there. Out of a lot of people that had close encounters, only three made it to the side of the mountain. Out of those three, only two made it over the mountain and beheld an awesome unexpected encounter with the UFOs. What makes so many people back off from their passion and dreams when they are so close?

"For many are called, but few are chosen" (Matthew 22:14, KJV). Don't let the wilderness experience detour you from your purpose. Learn from the situation and know that what you learn from the wilderness will catapult you forward. Stand your ground. "...and having done all, to stand" (Ephesians 6:14, KJV). When you have done all you can do, you have to let God do the rest. There is nothing else you can do. This is the exciting part. Because you are out of the way, God will do miracles on your behalf. Remember, He wants to get all the honor, glory, and praise!

The healing process is where the rubber meets the road. You will learn who you are and what you are made of. How firm is your foundation? How deep are your roots? You will learn during this process. You need to speak the word of God and hear the word. I know that when you're injured this gets tricky because people could be around helping you. Make sure you have ear buds. So, you don't annoy them. There are so many resources to build your faith, teachings and Bible apps. The more you hear the word, the more you are building your faith up. "So, then faith comes by hearing, and hearing by the word of God" (Romans 10:17, KJV). "Now faith is the confidence in what we hope for, and assurance about what we do not see" (Hebrews 11:1).

Let me ask you: What are you hoping for? What do you need to move forward with your healing? What is your purpose on this earth? These are some questions that you will need to ask yourself and God. You will have to seek out the answers for yourself and dig deep within. During this time, you will learn a lot about yourself-some things you won't like about yourself and some stuff you will like. Deal with whatever is holding your back and let go of what doesn't serve you. Most of all, you will realize that you are stronger than you ever thought.

I would also encourage you to think about ways you can be the answer to someone else's problem. What if you are going through these injuries so you can help others when they get injured? I always felt that this was part of my purpose. I want to encourage people through the healing process because it's important to have people to lean on during this time. No one should go through this by themselves and you can offer your strength to others.

Mary Manin said, "Even though you may want to move forward in your life, you may have one foot on the brakes. To be free, we must learn how to let go. Release the hurt. Release the fear. Refuse to entertain your old pain. The energy it takes to hold onto the past is holding you back from a new life. What is it you would let go of today?"

Take a moment and really think about that. Sometimes we have to get over ourselves because "we" are the problem. If your head is down, you can't see the light at the end of the tunnel. You only see the problem. May I suggest that you start looking for the positive in your situation? I'm not saying pain is positive, but there is more to life than pain. I had to do this myself—I had to make the choice to stop dwelling on the pain even though it was constantly there. I had to choose to focus on the daily progress that I was making. One day, I realized I was finally off of my medication. Another day, I could get up by myself. Another day, I could fix my own food. I had to choose to focus on the "baby steps" of progress that I was making. The key is, don't look too far ahead. Focus on today and handle what you can do today.

If there is one thought I want you to take away from this chapter is: don't be so hard on yourself. Don't overlook this opportunity to slow down and pace yourself. Enjoy the downtime that you have. Focus on the fact that it will get better. Remember where you came from and what lessons you have learned on your journey so you can move forward and help others.

YOU ARE NOT ALONE

CHAPTER ELEVEN

Don't Hide Your Victories

"But thanks be to God, who always leads us as captives in Christ's triumphal procession and uses us to spread the aroma of the knowledge of him everywhere."

2 CORINTHIANS 2:14

How comfortable do you feel to talk about yourself to others? Are you open to sharing about your life's obstacles and what you've had to overcome to get where you are now? Or do you shy away from difficult topics because you think people won't accept you if they know about your struggles? Do you keep quiet instead?

Many people battle internal thoughts thinking that people won't want to hear what they have to say. Their thoughts make them feel small and insignificant. They think that their victory isn't a big deal. Or they somehow feel ashamed about what they've been delivered from. Some even doubt their healing and wonder if the pain or issue will come back. They feel that they are not good enough or strong enough to help others. They compare themselves to others and think, "Other people have better stories and bigger miracles."

If this is you, I want to tell you today to open your mouth and share your story! Someone needs to hear about your victory. Your story matters and it can mean the world to someone else. It starts by sharing with just one person, and then it turns into two, and then three. You never know how many people you can impact by sharing what you've been through. There is a song that states, "It only takes a spark to get a fire going. And soon all those around can warm up in its glowing." We need to spark others and inspire them to victory. You might not have your victory story yet, but it is coming!

As you share your victories, your realm of influence is expanded. New opportunities will open up for you to share about overcoming struggles. When you see the impact you have on people, you will be inspired to share more. Amazing things can happen in people's lives with or without pain. You already have tools inside of you that God has placed there, and He will make sure you're given opportunities to minister to those who are hurting like you were.

"They triumphed over him by the blood of the Lamb and by the word of their testimony..." (Revelation 12:11).

Wherever you go, you can minister life and encouragement to people. You have no idea what the people you encounter each day are going through—people at the grocery store, post office, or anywhere you are out. Look for their individuality and value the uniqueness of people. God does. Everyone needs love and encouragement to get through their obstacles just like you did. You never know how God will cause your path to cross the right person at the right time who needs to hear your story.

Why is a testimony so powerful? A testimony speaks of evidence. What is evidence? Evidence is defined by the available body of facts or information indicating whether a belief or proposition is true or valid. When you share your testimony, you are telling people that you have actual proof that God does what He says He will do. You can trust Him. You actually prove to others that you got through painful situations in your life. Not only that but you are the evidence! You are the proof. A lot of times people will even ask what did you do to accomplish this? You can then explain what you had to do to become an overcomer.

So, pick up your spiritual sword for battle and poke and take stabs at your situation. I've seen so many prophetic demonstrations using a sword. This is the sword of the spirit that will bring down strongholds in your life or things that have held you captive. No more! Rise up and fight your battle! No one can fight your battle, but you. You have to war with the word of God and your testimony, but the good news is--you will win! With God on your side, all things are possible.

Because I've gone through so many surgeries with my feet, I have become sensitive to the pain of others with foot injuries. I know the struggles that they have encountered and will encounter because of it. When I meet an individual with a boot on their foot or using a walker with wheels (Squeaky-the name of my walker), or using crutches, immediately I must approach them to ask about their story. I take time for them and let them know about my story and how I got through. Normally, I'm rushing all over the place. Running errands here and there trying to get them done as fast as possible. My friends can and will attest to this. They see me on the highway very focused to get from Point A to Point B. I'll find out later that they were waving to me as they passed by and I was not paying any attention to them. However, when I see someone in a situation that I used to be in, my life comes to a screeching halt. In an instant, I will make time for that person. They need someone to comfort them and relate to what they are going through. They want someone to understand that the pain they feel is not in their head. I want them to understand that though they are injured for a while, they still are valuable. Their life counts. They will get through this. How do I know? Because I got through it. If I can get through it, everyone will get through it.

Not everyone you share with will understand and connect with your experience. That's why I want to encourage you to look for people who are dealing with the same type of pain as you went through. Not that you want to have a pity party together but you can encourage each other because you have that common experience. But, don't stop there. Yes, you have a common problem, but you know who has the answer to solve your problem! You can't solve it by yourself. This is why there are so many support groups. They get a group of people that have to deal with the same problem and bring them into a meeting. Not to flaunt them or laugh at them. But, to encourage, and let them have a comfortable place to share their pain. They will help each other overcome the pain in their life.

Share Your Scars

As with any battle or war, there will be scars. They might be hidden or visible, but they are there. I know because I have them. I have a titanium rod to straighten my big toe, a plate and screws on both ends that surround a bone graft. This is my scar from war. I always tell people that an x-ray of my foot looks like a table with four chairs. I compare it to several scriptures that says, "You prepare a table before me in the presence of my enemies. You anoint my head with oil; my cup overflows" (Psalm 23:5). "The Lord says to my Lord: Sit at my right hand until I make your enemies a footstool for your feet" (Psalm 110:1). My foot is scriptural! I have a physical reminder that my enemies are a footstool for my feet. "The God of peace will soon crush Satan under your feet" (Romans 16:20). These scriptures have given me such comfort even through all the years of dealing with constant physical pain. I will use my feet to move forward in the authority and power of God in any situation or battle that comes my way. Not because of my strength but because of His.

When I do see people in a situation that I have faced, it reminds me of what I've come through. Four surgeries are a lot of surgeries. Each one was for a particular reason. I didn't feel it at the time, but, looking back it kept me moving in the right direction. I had people in my life who loved me. I had friends that would call and keep in touch. I remember before one of my surgeries, my best friend gave me a pair of pointe shoes. No, I wasn't en pointe. No, I wasn't going to dance in them. She gave them to me as a tangible reminder of why the surgeries were necessary in my life. I would be reminded of my passion for dance every time I saw them. Her thoughtfulness worked. What an awesome friend to have. I still have them and use them for decorations at the ticket tables for ballet shows. Through the years people have asked to buy them, but they are not for sale. But, every time I bring them out, I'm reminded of my past and how it helped me to get through.

Was the pain of surgery worth it? Was the pain of going through physical therapy worth it? It was worth it if I can encourage just one person who needs to know that someone made it and they can too. It was all worth it. God is true to His word, He convinced me that this pain I was suffering was not about me. I thought it was. It felt like it was. But in the end, it wasn't. God wanted to show out. God needed someone to show how strong He was. That vessel was me. God needed me. God wants to get all the glory, honor, and praise. There is no way that I could have gotten through those surgeries relying on my own strength. I had none. I knew that I had none. There was none to be found. I have a high tolerance of pain; that's about all I can say. God did the rest.

Going through the pain has humbled me as well as has slowed my life down to a simmer. OK, maybe a fast simmer. I know I have a testimony that is powerful to help people overcome pain with regards to surgeries with feet. Remember, you will have power and authority with whatever you have had to overcome. I can't say that I can help all people with all kinds of pain. No, just the pain that I have had to deal with and got to the other side, if you will. I've heard the quote, "Without any test there is no "mony." Your testimony is what defines you, not your past. There is power in your tongue. Use it for God's glory and not idle words.

We will experience some type of pain in our lives. I'm not prophesying pain on anybody's life. I'm just stating a fact. If you live on the earth long enough something is going to come your way that is going to cause you pain. There is a way to live through the pain. So many stories are out there of heroes helping other people. People like stories. People need to hear your story.

The Gift of Pain

As this book comes to a close, I want to leave with you a couple of things. I was on Facebook one time and saw a segment of the Ellen DeGeneres show. She was interviewing the singer, Pink. She stated, "Inspiration comes from pain. Creativity gets us out of painful situations. Pain catapults for change. Does art come from happiness? "No." After which, Ellen exclaimed, "You should try pain." Of course, everyone laughed, but there is a lot of truth to that statement. You will go much farther when you deal with pain in your life. I'm not saying that you should go after it, but you will learn a lot about yourself. More so than if you didn't have any pain at all.

"No one changes unless they want to. Not if you beg them. Not if you shame them. Not if you use reason, emotion or tough love. There's only one thing that makes someone change: their own realization that they need to do it..." (Lori Deschene) This is so true. You can't make any one do anything. They have to want it for themselves. They have to make the decision to change their situation. When they make up their mind to change, they will change. Many times, I have heard of stories where people woke up and decided, "Today I'm going to start exercising." You know what? They lost a lot of weight. They saw something in their life that needed changing and did something about it. Others start tweaking their diet. They make lifestyle changes that affect their outlook on life. It all started happening with one thought. They said enough is enough. What do I have to do to change? They change. Others see that they changed and they want to change.

As I spend time with God, poems, or songs often come to me. This song was from Psalm 56:9:

> Because God is for me
>
> In God (I will praise His Word)
>
> In the Lord (I will praise His Word)
>
> In God, (I will put my trust)
>
> I will not be afraid.

I haven't mentioned anything about fear yet, but fear is real. There are many scriptures in the Bible about fear—scriptures that tell us not to fear! If there are a lot of scriptures telling us not to fear then we need to grasp the concept and choose not to fear. There are a lot of things we can be afraid of. We are afraid of the unknown because there is a risk involved here. Are we going to step out on a limb and take the risk that God is God? He knows what we need, when we need it. He already knows what we are going through and He has a plan to bring us through.

My prayer for you is that you don't get stuck and think your life is over because you are dealing with pain in your life or that your life is never going to get better. Know that you are capable of so much more. Reach for the stars. Expect more and you will get more. Take one step at a time. Each step that you make is progress. Remember the story of the hare and the tortoise? Everyone thought that the hare was going to win. However, the hare didn't win. The tortoise was slow and steadily moving forward and focused on what was before him. The tortoise was determined to keep the course. He had limitations, but he didn't let his limitations stop him from moving forward.

Don't let pain stop you from achieving your dreams no matter how slowly you are going. It's all up to you and your perspective. You can stay focused and accomplish great things in spite of your pain. Rise up and embrace the eminent victory. Moving forward in spite of the pain—this is the tortoise effect and remember the tortoise always wins!

About the Author

Juanita M. Clendaniel is a native Delawarean and resides in Milford, Delaware. She did live in Tulsa, Oklahoma for nine years; but, moved back to be with family.

She has two Bachelor of Science degrees: Business Administration and Music Education (piano was her major medium). She enjoys sewing, playing/practicing multiple instruments, singing and dancing.

Juanita is currently an elementary music teacher in the Cape Henlopen School District in Lewes, Delaware.

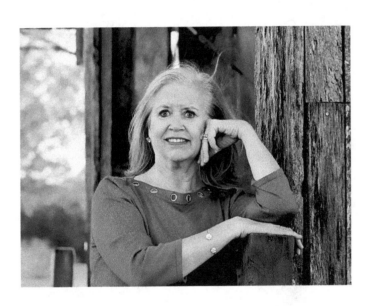